AF307215

Raul J. Rosenthal   Richard L. Friedman
Edward H. Phillips (Eds.)

The Pathophysiology of Pneumoperitoneum

Springer

Berlin
Heidelberg
New York
Barcelona
Budapest
Hong Kong
London
Milan
Paris
Santa Clara
Singapore
Tokyo

Raul J. Rosenthal
Richard L. Friedman
Edward H. Phillips (Eds.)

The Pathophysiology
of Pneumoperitoneum

With 51 Figures and 14 Tables

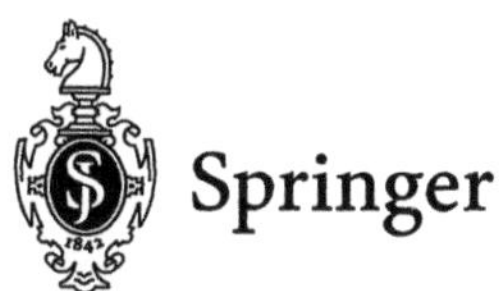

Springer

Raul J. Rosenthal M.D.
Department of Surgery
Mount Sinai Medical Center
The Mount Sinai Hospital
Mount Sinai School of Medicine
One L. Gustave Levy Place
New York, NY 10029-6574, USA

Richard L. Friedman M.D.
Beth Israel Medical Center
Department of Surgery
16th Street and 1st. Ave
New York, NY 10002, USA

Edward H. Phillips, M.D., F.A.C.S.
Division of Endoscopic Surg.
Cedars-Sinai Medical Center
8700 Beverly Boulevard
Los Angeles, CA 90048, USA

ISBN-13:978-3-642-64339-2

Cataloging-in-Publication Data applied for

The pathophysiology of pneumoperitoneum: with tabels/ Raul J. Rosenthal ... (ed.). – Berlin; Heidelberg; New York; Barcelona; Budapest; Hong Kong; London; Milan; Paris; Santa Clara; Singapore; Tokyo: Springer, 1998
  ISBN-13:978-3-642-64339-2   e-ISBN-13:978-3-642-60290-0
  DOI: 10.1007/978-3-642-60290-0

Typesetting: Michael Kusche, Goldener Schnitt

SPIN: 10554611   24/3135 – 5 4 3 2 1 0 – Printed on acid-free paper

In Memoriam Karl Storz, 1911–1996

Dr. Karl Storz was born in Tuttlingen, Germany and established his own company in 1945 specializing in ENT instrumentation. Throughout his career, he worked in close collaboration with surgeons to develop practical, precise, and well-engineered instrumentation. His imagination revolutionized the industry. He developed binocular magnification, direct and indirect laryngoscopes and bronchoscopes, video choledochoscopy, and shock-proof ceramic arc light bulb illumination. When Dr. Storz was introduced to the Hopkins rod lens system, he quickly adapted the technology to medicine offering us instrumentation with superb light transmission and a superior image.

He was an individual with very rare characteristics. He was absolutely honest. He was generous to his community and deservedly his friends, and was a wonderful father and family man. He received many awards throughout his career, but was especially proud when he was awarded an honorary doctorate degree from the Universtiy of Marburg in 1985. Also, he was the first to receive the Pioneer in Endoscopy Award from the American Society of Gastrointestinal Endoscopic Surgeons.

With all of these wonderful accomplishments, those who knew him remember him most for his sense of humor and compassion. We all admire him for his commitment to the advancement of medicine through endoscopy.

EDWARD H. PHILLIPS, RAUL J. ROSENTHAL

Dedication

To my wife Simona and our children Dana and Noam

Raul J. Rosenthal

To my father, Ira H. Friedman MD "A Surgeons Surgeon", for his life-long teaching and his moral and academic example.

My mother for her love and her tireless and endless support.
My wife Cheryl and my children Shoshana, Elana, Adina, Tzippora and Shmuel Aryeh for all their loving support and understanding, especially during the times I have not been there.

Richard L. Friedman

To my wife, Nancy, my children, Aaron, Rachel and David.

To my father, who was my first physiology teacher and,

To Dr. Leonard Rosoff, past Chairman, Department of Surgery, University of Southern California, who taught me to be a doctor, a scientist and a student.

To Dr. Achilles Demetriou, Chairman of Surgery, Cedars Sinai Medical Center Los Angeles, who exemplifies the scientist surgeon.

Edward H. Phillips

Foreword

For the safe and efficient performance of every operative procedure it is necessary to have adequate access and optimal exposure. Discovered serendipitously, es the initial chapter on history notes, pneumoperitoneum, most commonly obtained with insufflation of carbon dioxide, has permitted the visceral separation required for the performance of most laparoscopic surgery. While laparoscopists of various disciplines have learned the technical aspects of its performance, and recently, there has been little information available on its pathophysiological affects. This is not surprising since the laparoscopy has, for many years, mainly performed been for diagnostic purposes. With the introduction and rapid expansion of operative laparoscopy, the limitations and morbidity of carbon dioxide pneumoperitoneum have spurred useful investigation into how it works, what its limitations are and how they may be modified. The editors of this monograph are to be congratulated for undertaking what is clearly the most exhaustive review of pneumoperitoneum at a time when the technique itself is being challenged by alternative methods of visceral separation. By studying the physiologic consequences of pneumoperitoneum in such detail, a standard has truly been not, against which future modifications or substitutions for pneumoperitoneum will doubtless be measured. Since many feel that the advantage of pneumoperitoneum my be sustained but that the type of gas insufflated has to be less hindered by morbidity (as in carbon dioxide), the physiologic effects of other gasses are explained in detail to the extent to which they have been studied.

By choosing experts (incidently, from widely separated geographic regione) not only in laparoscopy but also in their chosen specialities of surgery, the reader is given more authoritative insight into the physiologic effects which genuinely matter in clinical practice. Particularly useful are the chapters that deal with special situations such as pediatric age and pregnancy and the discussion of anesthetic techniques. The various chapters not only review the individual subjects in depth but also provide the reader with detailed analysis of the evidence from basic science, live models, and clinical studies with up-to-date bibliographies. One of the advantages of selecting experts carefully for the writing of book chapters is that the reader can be provided not only with historical and state-of-the-art perspectives, but the equally important dimension of identifying areas in need of further study. As the field of minimal access surgery expands, as we operate on patients at higher risk, we need to recognize not only the complex changes associated with pneumoperitoneum but also how to avoid or manage them. As various sophisticated cardiac, respiratory and other monitoring systems are now more widely available, knowledge of their integration into minimal access surgery will allow for safer and more efficient patient management. Details of these issues are well covered in this work.

KENNETH A. FORDE

Contents

List of Contributors

ANDRUS, CHARLES H., M.D., F.A.C.S., Assoc. Professor of Surgery
Hines Veterans Administration Medical Center,
2160 South First Avenue, Maywodd, IL 60153, USA

AZAR, ISAAC, M.D., Assoc. Prof. of Anesthesiology
Department of Anesthesiology,
Beth Israel Medical Center New York,
Albert Einstein College of Medicine, 16th Street (off 1st Avenue),
New York, NY 10003, USA

BERCI, GEORGE, M.D., F.A.C.S. hon. F.R.C.S., Assoc. Prof. of Surgery
University of Southern California,
Cedars Sinai Medical Center, 8700 Beverly Boulevard,
Los Angeles, CA 90048, USA

BESSELL, JUSTIN R., M.D., M.B.B.S, F.R.A.C.S
University of Adelaide Department of Surgery,
The Queen Elizabeth Hospital, Woodville,
South Australia 5011, Australia

BOCKHORN, HERMANN, M.D., Ph.D. Professor
Department of Surgery,
Johann Wolfgang Goethe University,
Nordwest Krankenhaus, Steinbacher Hohl 2–26,
D-60488 Frankfurt am Main, Germany

CHRISTEN, YVES, M.D.
Division of Angiology and Hemostasis,
University Hospital of Geneva, Case Postale,
CH 1211, Geneve 14, Switzerland

CORWIN, CLAUDIA, M.D.
Department of Surgery and Transplantation,
University of Iowa Hospitals and Clinics,
Iowa City, IA 52242 – 1086, USA

DAVIS, MICHAEL G., M.D.
University of Montreal,
Director of Pulmonary Function Laboratory,
Montreal Children's Hospital, 2300 Tupper, Room D380,
Montreal, Quebec, Canada

DIEBEL, LAWRENCE N., M.D., Assoc. Professor of Surgery
Wayne State University School of Medicine,
University Health Center 6C,
4201 St. Antoine Street, Detroit, MI 48201, USA

DENNHARDT, RÜDIGER, Professor Dr. med
Department of Anesthesia
Nordwest Krankenhaus
Steinbacher Hohl 2–26
D-60488 Frankfurt am Main, Germany

ELEFTHERIADIS, EFTHIMIOS, M.D., Professor of Surgery
Department of Surgery,
Aristotelian University of Thessaloniki Medical School,
54006 Thessaloniki, Greece

FABREGA, ALFREDO J., M.D.
Department of Surgery and Transplantation,
University of Iowa Hospitals and Clinics,
Iowa City, IA 52242 – 1086, USA

FILIPI, CHARLES J., M.D., F.A.C.S., Professor of Surgery
Department of Surgery,
Creighton University, 601 N 30th Street,
Omaha, NE 68131, USA

FORDE, KENNETH A., MD, Professor of Surgery
Columbia Prebyterian Medical Center
Department of Surgery
161 Fr. Washington Ave.,
New York, NY. 10032

FRIEDMAN, RICHARD L., M.D.
Albert Einstein School of Medicine
Coordinator Advanced Laparoscopic Surgery
Beth Israel Medical Center New York, 16th Street and 1st Ave.
New York, NY 10002, USA

GREENE, FREDERICK L., M.D., F.A.C.S., Professor of Surgery
University of South Carolina School of Medicine,
Columbia, SC, USA

JAKUB, JAMES, M.D., F.A.C.S.
Department of Surgery,
Richland Memorial Hospital, University of South Carolina
School of Medicine,
Columbia, South Carolina, USA

KAMINSKY, DONALD L., M.D., F.A.C.S., Professor of Surgery
Department of General Surgery,
St. Louis University Hospital, 3635 Vista Avenue,
St. Louis, MO 63110 – 0250, USA

KOCKERLING, FERDINAND, M.D., Professor
Department of Surgery,
University of Erlangen-Nürnberg,
Postfach 3560, D-91023 Erlangen, Germany

KOTZAMPASSI, KATHERINA, M.D.
Department of Surgery,
Aristotelian University of Thessaloniki Medical School,
54006 Thessaloniki, Greece

LACY, ANTONIO M., M.D., Ph.D.
Department of Surgery,
University Hospital of Barcelona,
Villarroel 170, 08036, Barcelona, Spain

LAUREANO, BEVERLY A., M.D.
Department of Surgery,
St. Louis University Hospital, 3635 Vista Avenue,
St. Louis, MO 63110 – 0250, USA

LOWHAM, ANTHONY S., M.D.
Department of Surgery,
Creighton University,
 601 N 30th Street, Omaha, NE 68131, USA

MADDERN, GUY J., M.D., M.B.B.S., F.R.A.C.S., M.S., Ph.D.,
Professor of Surgery
University of Adelaide Department of Surgery,
The Queen Elizabeth Hospital, Woodville,
South Australia 5011, Australia

MARTZ, JOSEPH, M.D.
Department of Surgery, Beth Israel Medical Center,
Albert Einstein School of Medicine, 16 th Street (off 1st Avenue),
New York, NY 10003, USA

MOREL, PHILLIPE, M.D.
Department of Digestive Surgery,
University Hospital of Geneva,
Case Postale, CH 1211, Geneve 14, Switzerland

PHILLIPS, EDWARD H., M.D., F.A.C.S., Assoc. Professor of Surgery
Director, Division of Endoscopic Surgery,
Associate clinical Professor
University of Southern California
Cedars Sinai Medical Center,
8635 W. 3rd Street, 785W, Los Angeles, CA 90048, USA

PLATT, LAWRENCE, M.D., Professor of Gyneaology
Department of Obsterics and Gynecology,
Cedars Sinai Medical Center, UCLA School of Medicine,
8700 Beverly Boulevard, Los Angeles, CA 90048, USA

REYMOND, MARC A., M.D.
Digestiva Surgery Clinic,
University Hospital of Geneva,
Case Postale, CH 1211, Geneve 14, Switzerland

ROSENTHAL, RAUL J., M.D.
Department of Surgery,
Mount. Sinai Medical Center,
The Mount Sinai Hospital,
Mount Sinai School of Medicine.
One L. Gustave Levy Place, New York, NY 10029–6574, USA

RUBIN, STEVEN Z., M.D., Professor of Pediatric Surgery
Department of Surgery, University of Ottawa,
Children's Hospital of Eastern Ontario,
Ottawa, Ontario, Canada K 1H8L1

SALA-BLANCH, XAVIER, M.D.
Department of Anesthesiology,
University Hospital of Barcelona,
Villarroel 170, 08036 Barcelona, Spain

SCOTT-CONNER, CAROL, M.D., Ph.D., Professor of Surgery
Department of Surgery and Transplantation,
University of Iowa College of Medicine,
200 Hawkins Drive, 1516 JCP, Iowa City,
IA 52242 – 1086, USA

SHIMIZU, MASAFUMI, M.D.
Department of Surgery II,
University Hospital, National Defense Medical College,
3–2 Namiki, Tokorozawa, Saitama 359, Japan

SILVA, JANA K., M.D.
Department of Obstetrics and Gynecology,
Division of Maternal Fetal Medicine,
Cedars Sinai Medical Center, UCLA School of Medicine,
8700 Beverly Boulevard, Los Angeles, CA 90048, USA

STEIGERWALD, SABINE, M.D.
Department of Surgery, Nordwest Krankenhaus,
Steinbacher Hohl 2–26, D-60488 Frankfurt am Main, Germany

TOMONAGA, TOMONAGA, M.D.
Department of Surgery,
Creighton University,
601 N 30th Street, Omaha, NE 68131, USA

VISA, JOSEP, M.D., Ph.D.
Department of Surgery,
University Hospital of Barcelona,
Villarroel 170, 08036 Barcelona, Spain

1 History of Pneumoperitoneum

G. BERCI

It is not uncommon for inventions to have been created for certain applications and then later employed for different purposes. Pneumoperitoneum is a case in point.

Before the turn of the century (1890), George Kelling (Fig. 1), a German surgeon, was interested in gastric physiology. He attempted to develop a technique to assess the size of the stomach. He introduced double balloons into the stomach and in the course of the experiment observed that the pressure in the abdominal cavity changed with the increase in gastric distention. He performed numerous experiments in animals and then went on to measure stomach displacements in 70 patients. He was quite inventive and when he later turned to the topic of endoscopic examination of the esophagus and stomach, he developed a flexible, tubular esophagoscope. It consisted of several joints hooked together by wires. If he pulled the wires and the tube was in a bent position, it could be straightened out. It was similar in structure to present-day neurosurgi-

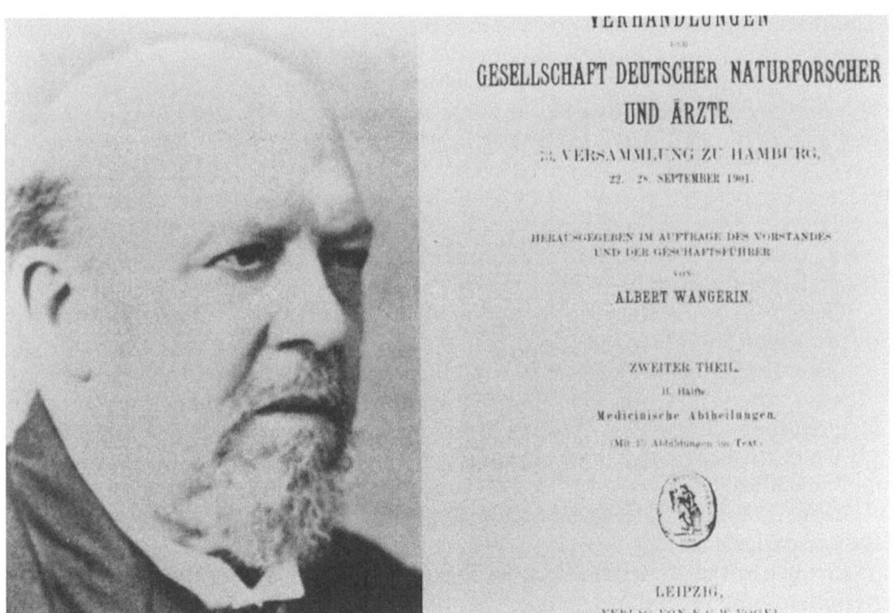

Fig. 1. George Kelling, M.D.

cal retractors consisting of a flexible arm which can be bent and then fixed in position by stretching wires. This esophagoscope was important because of the way he performed esophagoscopy. He started with the patient in a sitting position on a table. Dr. Kelling stepped onto a small step and introduced the esophagoscope in a bent position. The patient was then placed in a supine position with a hyperextended head which was held by an assistant, and the esophagoscope was straightened.

At the beginning of this century, Kelling became interested in the treatment of gastric hemorrhage and induced a pneumoperitoneum to apply pressure on the bleeding organ. In this way he hoped that abdominal tamponade would arrest the bleeding. He called this process "coelioseopy." He postulated that by increasing the intra-abdominal pressure to 50–60 mm of mercury (mmHg) he could achieve hemostasis.

Kelling tested this procedure on 20 experimental animals (dogs). The animals were anesthetized. While the intraabdominal pressure was increased, he measured the arterial pressure in the femoral and carotid arteries. He found that the femoral pressure remained the same while the carotid pressure increased by 10%. If only Kelling had measured the venous pressures as well! He asked two patients with upper intestinal bleeding to allow him to perform a pneumoperitoneum for hemostasis purposes but both refused.

In 1901, he wrote for the first time that intra-abdominal organs could be observed by introducing a trocar after the pneumoperitoneum was created and advancing a cystoscope for observation. In 1923, Kelling recommended that gastroscopy be performed by a direct percutaneous approach facilitated by a pneumoperitoneum and a small incision on the left side of the lateral edge of the rectus muscle. The stomach could then be grasped and incised and the gastroscope introduced. Needless to say, this approach did not find many followers [1–4].

In 1911, Jacobeus (Fig. 2) in Stockholm published his initial results using laparoscopy and thoracoscopy for diagnostic purposes. He described the pneumoperitoneum as a first step by performing laparoscopy. Kelling, who actually never used pneumoperitoneum as a laparoscopic technique, claimed priority and started a debate with Jacobeus in peer-reviewed journals. Jacobeus had already published a large series of patient case studies with very good results. It is interesting that even at the turn of the century the reader faced this question of "ego," which is not unheard of, even in the laparoscopic era of today [5].

There were sporadic reports of attempts to examine the abdominal cavity via pneumoperitoneum. In 1911, Berheim at John Hopkins Hospital examined two patients, inserting a small proctoscope through the abdominal wall. He called it organoscopy [6]. In 1911, Fervers used oxygen and CO_2 but turned to room air for pneumoperitoneum. Zollikofer from Switzerland preferred CO_2 to room air [7]. Thus, the debate as to what should be used as an insufflating agent goes back eight decades.

In 1924, Steiner, recommended laparoscopy with pneumoperitoneum after limited experience [8].

In the United States in 1937, Ruddock (an internist) was a proponent of peritoncoscopy (terminology used before WWI in the United States) [9]. He employed room air in 500 cases with a mortality rate of 0.2% [1].

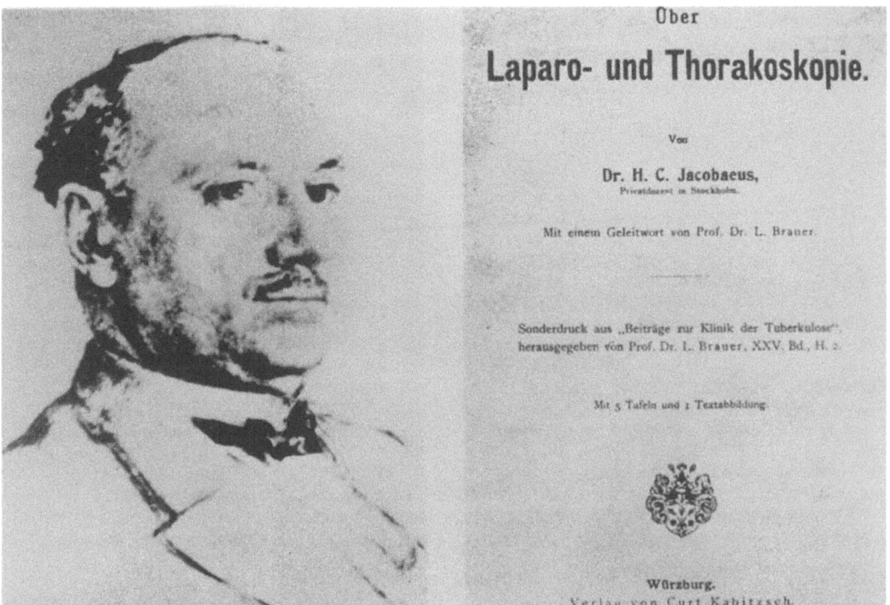

Fig. 2. H.C. Jacobeus, M.D.

However, the German gastroenterologist Kalk (Fig. 3) was the real pioneer. He introduced many new instruments and ideas on how to apply a safe pneumoperitoneum (Kalk 1929). He produced excellent data and the best documentation. He used a trocar with a spring-loaded stylet. The stylet jumped back into the trocar as soon as the abdominal cavity was entered. He introduced the 30° oblique viewing telescope and the dual trocar approach. The procedure was performed under sedation and local anesthesia. He was the first to recommend that the pneumoneedle be introduced in the left lower quadrant in ascitic patients. He recommended turning the needle immediately parallel to the abdominal wall to avoid creating air bubbles in the ascitic fluid, which can never be eliminated but can interfere with the examination [10].

Kalk had tremendous influence on the widespread use of laparoscopy in Europe, mainly among hepatologists because of the precise selection of the site on the liver for biopsy. He used room air exclusively for pneumoperitoneum. A normal standard rubber bulb (used for sphygmomanometers or rectoscopes) was employed. A little metal container was inserted into the tube, connecting the rubber bulb with the pneumo needle in which cotton wool was placed to filter air. Of course, there were no bacteriological data available, but, interestingly, these pioneers did not report any severe generalized or localized abdominal infections after air insufflation [11].

For several decades air insufflation was the method of choice. It was cheap and available. There was no downside as hepatologists mainly just performed

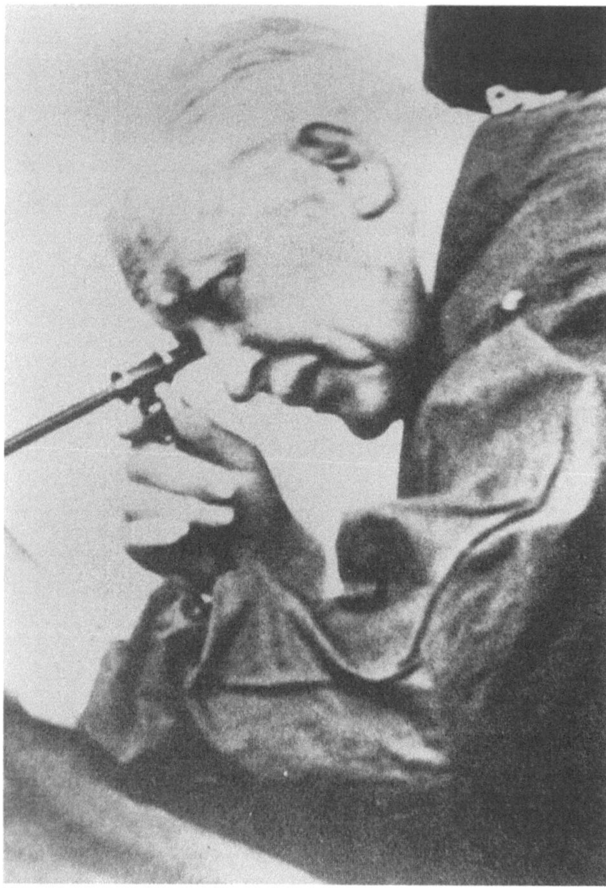

Fig. 3.   Hans Kalk, M.D.

needle biopsies (aspiration or Menghini type) where bleeding was minimal and could be arrested by compression. Gas embolisms were rare but existed [12,13].

It may be assumed that many air emboli cases were not reported. This is one of the reasons why when gynecologists became so interested in this subject and began using electrocoagulation, the preferred gas became CO_2, which was not combustible.

In 1938, a very important adjunct to pneumoperitoneum was the introduction of a spring-loaded blunt stylet type of needle with a side hole by Veress, a thoracic surgeon from Hungary. This needle (in its variations) became the needle of choice to perform a safe penetration of the abdominal wall [14]. Recently, the "open" technique has become popular, especially in the operated abdomen, to secure a safe gas insufflation for the abdominal cavity.

Since laparoscopy became widely accepted in gynecology and, in the past 7 years in general surgery, the simple manual insufflators previously available are no longer adequate to handle the longer operating times and flow requirements with multiple trocars and instrument exchanges. Most modern insufflators can supply 10 l of CO_2 per minute.

In this age there are many bells and whistles available to create a pneumoperitoneum. The high volume insufflator PAGE MARK, a built-in alarm signal to exchange the gas cylinder to have pre-warmed CO_2 insufflation, are all further ideas. In the use of video laparoscopy in minimally invasive procedures there is one interesting aspect which would be important during pneumoperitoneum induction, as well as during the entire procedure where an optimal pneumoperitoneum pressure should be continuously maintained: the display of the intra-abdominal pressure on a TV screen. The insufflators are hidden behind the assistants or behind the operating physician, and if there are changes it is difficult to recognize them in time. For instance, if there is a leak and loss of pressure somewhere, then we recognize this phenomenon only after our working area collapses and we cannot see anything. It is very easy for the human eye to inspect a corner, as well as to observe the middle of the TV screen. If the pressure drops by a few millimeters of mercury it can be recognized immediately and the time loss caused by finding out where the leakage is, etc., can be avoided.

Various gases have been employed in the past [15]. As described in other chapters, even with all its disadvantages, CO_2 is still the most preferred and economically feasible choice for creating a pneumoperitoneum.

Without elevating the abdominal wall and creating a working space for the surgeon's manipulations, there is no chance that laparoscopic surgery would ever have been accepted, least of all in the abdominal cavity. From the early stages of room air insufflation the pendulum has swung rapidly towards the use of CO_2. It absorbs well, while small amounts injected intravascularly do not cause fatal air emboli (only a minor incidence of latter). Carbon dioxide has become the gas of choice for the creation of pneumoperitoneum. Side effects that can occur in the

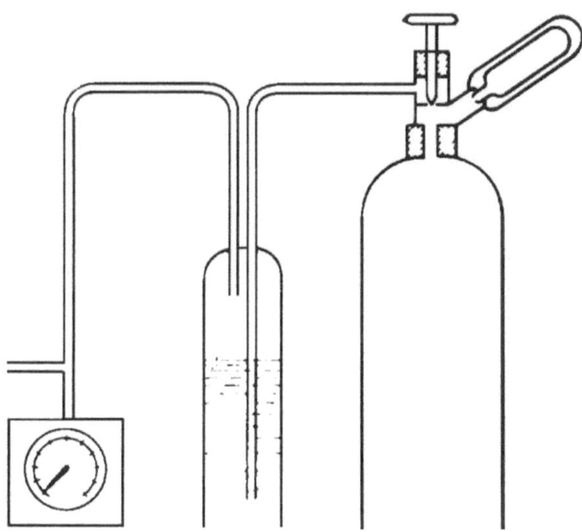

Fig. 4. Standard CO_2 canister with pressure gauge

hemodynamic status can be compensated for by the skill of the anesthesiologist and that of the surgeon using lower pressure. Some patients complain of shoulder pain for a day or so, which can be well compensated by analgesics. There is hyperemia visible on the vessels of the intestinal scrosa, but overall, taking other agents into consideration (helium, etc.), CO_2 is the most efficient and the least expensive.

Attempts were made to lift the abdominal wall with two towel clips and introduce the trocar without pneumoperitoneum, but this "safe" technique failed because of the high incidence of intestinal perforations. We have come a long way, moving from room air insufflation to the use of simple CO_2 canisters or soda cartridges (Fig. 4) and now, in recent years, to the use of electronically controlled insufflators. Pneumoperitoneum is our working horse to create space and to facilitate telescopic observation and the introduction of manipulatory instruments. If it is employed carefully, it is a safe agent for laparoscopy.

References

1. Kelling G (1890) Uber die Ermittelung der Magengroesse. Reichel, Dresden
2. Kelling G (1901) Die Tamponade der Bauchhoehle mit Luft zur Stillung lebensgefaehrlicher Intestinalblutungen. Munch Med Wochenschr 48: 1480–1535
3. Kelling G (1910) Uber die Moglichkeit, die Zystoskopic bei Untersuchung seroser Hoehlungen anzuwenden. Bemerkungen zu dem Artikel von Jacobaeus. Munch Med Wochenschr 57:2358
4. Litynski G, Schaeff B, Paolucci V (1996) Vom Pneumoperitoneum bis zur Koelioskopie. Chirurg 67:283–287
5. Jacobeus HC (1911) Kurze Ubersicht uber meine Erfahrungen mit der Laparoskopie. Munch Med Wochenschr 58:2017
6. Bemheim BM (1911) Organoscopy. Cystoscopy of the abdominal cavity. Ann Surg, 53:764
7. Fervers C (1933) Die Laparoskopie mit dem Zystoskope. Med Klin 19:1042
8. Steiner OP (1924) Abdominoskopie. Schweiz Med Wochschr 54:84
9. Ruddock JC (1937) Peritoneoscopy. Surg Gynecol Obstet 65:523
10. Kalk H (1929) Erfahrungen mit der Laparoskopie. Z. Klin. Med 11 1:303–348
11. Kalk H, Bruhl W (1951) Leitfaden der Laparoskopie. Thieme, Stuttgart
12. Root B, Levy N, Pollack W, Lubert M, Pathak K (1978) Gas embolism death after laparoscopy delayed by "trapping" in portal circulation. Anesth Analg 57: 232–237
13. Cottlin V, Delafosse B, Viale JP (1996) Gas embolism during laparoscopy. Surg Endosc 10:166–169
14. Veress J (1938) Neues Instrument zur Ausfuhrung von Brust oder Bauchpunktionen und Pneumothoraxbehandlung. Dtsch Med Wochenschr 64:1480
15. Hunter JG, Staheli J, Oddsdottir M, Trus T (1995) Nitrous oxide pneumoperitoneum revisited. Surg Endosc 9:501–504

2 Alternative Gases in Laparoscopic Surgery

A. Lacy, X. Sala Blanch, and J. Visa

Introduction

Visualization within the peritoneal cavity requires space in which to emit light, receive the nonabsorbed light, and maneuver. In laparoscopic surgery this is accomplished by filling the peritoneal cavity with a gas that distends the abdominal wall. The history of laparoscopy is replete with efforts to use many different gases for establishing pneumoperitoneum, including room air, nitrous oxide, oxygen, and carbon dioxide. The ideal gas for pneumoperitoneum should be nontoxic, colorless, readily soluble in blood, easily ventilated through the lungs, nonflammable, and inexpensive. Carbon dioxide is the standard gas used for pneumoperitoneum. The reason for this is that both oxygen and air are not absorbed as readily and therefore are more likely to result in death if an air embolism occurs. Nitrous oxide is dangerous because of unpredictable and uncontrollable absorption into the bloodstream. Moreover, oxygen and nitrous oxide support combustion if mixed with methane and have been associated with instances of intra-abdominal explosion [1–4].

Carbon Dioxide

Carbon dioxide is relatively inert, permitting the use of electrocoagulation, and is readily absorbed by the peritoneal membrane. Current surgical practice is to use CO_2 since it is noncombustible and thus will not create an explosion should the electrocautery generate a spark or ignite bowel gas (methane/hydrogen). Carbon dioxide is colorless, highly soluble in blood with a solubility coefficient of 0.49 at 37°C (as compared to 0.013 for nitrogen), and is readily expired via the lungs. These properties have popularized the use of carbon dioxide for the induction and sustaining of pneumoperitoneum.

Side Effects of Carbon Dioxide

In laparoscopic operations the side effects of pneumoperitoneum are the result of coupling an increased intra-abdominal pressure with the use of carbon dioxide as the insufflation gas. Some of the pneumoperitoneum-related changes in hemodynamic parameters include increased systemic arterial and central venous pressures, increased systemic vascular resistance, and a drop in cardiac output.

Other major alterations such as central hypertension, arrhythmia, decreased mesenteric blood flow, hypercarbia, acidosis, and increased vasopresin release have all been documented [8–15].

Normal intra-abdominal pressure alone or carbon dioxide at low intra-abdominal pressures does not lead to changes in respiratory mechanics. The same applies to changes in the acid-base balance. Thus, systemic changes such as acidosis, increases in $PaCO_2$ and carbon dioxide production were attributable to the absorption and local effects of carbon dioxide on the peritoneal area. Significant hemodynamic effects are usually only achieved by a combination of both carbon dioxide and high intra-abdominal pressure [16].

Some complications of pneumoperitoneum are directly related to the mechanical effects associated with raised intra-abdominal pressure. In laparoscopic operations the effects of the pneumoperitoneum on the patient's cardiopulmonary condition have been described [10, 12, 14, 17–28]. These effects are the result of various changes at the mechanical, ventilatory, cellular, hormonal, and immunological levels [16, 28–33]. The increase in intraperitoneal volume and pressure caused by pneumoperitoneum restricts diaphragmatic movement with an increase in required peak pulmonary ventilation pressure and a reduction of pulmonary compliance [34]. Several authors have asserted that moderate increases in peritoneal pressure may be accompanied by an increased effective cardiac filling pressure and therefore an increased cardiac output. Ishizaki demonstrated no change in cardiac output below intra-abdominal pressures of 16 mmHg [29]. However, when the intraperitoneal pressure is higher than 30 cm H_2O, it significantly reduces blood flow in the inferior vena cava and reduces cardiac output.

The use of CO_2 for pneumoperitoneum produces significant elevations in serum CO_2 ($PaCO_2$) and end tidal CO_2 ($ETCO_2$) levels associated with a drop in serum pH levels This hypercarbia is primarily due to peritoneal absorption of CO_2 [14, 35, 36, 37, 38]. In healthy patients, the insufflation of intraperitoneal CO_2 causes clinically insignificant changes in CO_2 homeostasis. However, mild hypercarbia and an increase in measured CO_2 production in the splanchnic area can be detected. The arterial systemic effects can be counteracted by a mechanical hyperventilation support. However, the growth of CO_2 concentrations in local splanchnic tissue cannot be remedied with changes in the characteristics of mechanical ventilation (increased minute ventilation). This CO_2 local concentration is dependent upon a number of variables, including cellular metabolism, local tissue perfusion, and regional blood flow (impaired by high intra-abdominal pressure) [34]. In other patients with pre-existing cardiovascular dysfunction or pulmonary disturbances, the development of significant hypercarbia and acidemia cannot be corrected without cessation of the pneumoperitoneum. Hypercarbia may produce significant increases in systolic blood pressure and heart rate. This shortens the pre-ejection period and left ventricular ejection time, and it shortens the diastolic filling phase of the coronary arteries [33]. Table 1 summarizes the effects of intra-abdominal pressure and hypercarbia on cardiovascular and hemodynamic parameters.

Hypercarbia also causes sympathetic nervous system stimulation as demonstrated by increases in plasma catecholamine levels [36]. Animal data suggest

Table 1. Effects of high intra-abdominal pressure (HIAP) and hypercarbia on hemodynamic parameters, regional blood flow, and ventilatory status

	IAP	Hypercarbia Local effect	Systemic effect
Hemodynamic Effects			
HR	↑ =	=	↑
CO	↓ =	↓↓	↑↑
MAP	↑ =	↓	↑↑
MPAP	↑	↑↑	↑
CVP	↑	↓	↑
PWP	↑	↑	↑
SVR	↑	↓	↓
PVR	↑	↑↑	↑
Splanchnic blood flow	↓↓↓	↑↑↑	↓
Renal blood flow	↓	↑↑	↓
Adrenal gland blood flow	↑=	↑↑	↓
Ventilatory parameters			
Peak airway pressure	↑	=	=
Pulmonary compliance	↓	=	=
Vital capacity	↓	=	=
Functional residual capacity	↓	=	=
Intrathoracic pressure	↑	=	=

HR, heart rate (beat/min); CO, cardiac output (l/min); MAP, mean arterial blood pressure (mmHg); MPAP, mean pulmonary arterial pressure (mmHG); CVP, central venous pressure (mm HG); PWP, pulmonary wedge pressure (mm HG); SVR, systemic vascular resistance (dyne s/cm^5); PVR, pulmonary vascular resistance (dyne s/cm^5).

that increased intra-abdominal pressure, not stress by itself, releases arginine vasopressin (AVP) via a reflex involving visceral pain receptors and the posterior spinal nerve roots. A fivefold increase in plasma AVP was recorded in 50% of patients in relation with the combination of high intra-abdominal pressure and CO_2 pneumoperitoneum. High abdominal pressure with a concomitant release of AVP has the potential of inducing functional impairment in abdominal organs and tissues. Caldwell et al. [39] proved in their experimental study that elevated intra-abdominal pressure (more than 20 mmHg) caused a decrease in organ blood flow index for all organs (abdominal and retroperitoneal) except the renal cortex and the adrenal gland. These changes are more significant than what the fall in cardiac output alone can account for, suggesting local control mechanisms. Intra-abdominal pressure associated with high levels of AVP probably reduce hepatic and intestinal oxygenation with a reduction in portal blood flow [40], as well as renal vein blood flow.

Our study group demonstrated that high intraperitoneal pressure in prolonged laparoscopic procedures causes a significant metabolic acidosis in relation to increased lactate levels. During long-lasting laparoscopic procedures, plasmatic lactate levels could be related to impairment of the regional tissue oxygenation/

perfusion ratio with the development of anaerobic metabolism [41]. Volz et al. [16] concluded in a recent paper that a reduction in intra-abdominal pressure with the use of carbon dioxide as the insufflation gas should result in normal acid-base balance. These authors suggest the importance of local effects due to a combination of intraperitoneal pressure, type of gas used, and duration of the application. The unfavorable changes in acid–base balance could be related to the result of peritoneal release chemotactic factors such as mediators by endotoxin. There is theoretical concern that the use of laparoscopy in conditions complicated by peritonitis may worsen the outcome. However, in a ground-breaking published paper based on an animal model of peritonitis, the authors concluded that there is no difference between pneumoperitoneum and laparotomy with respect to bacteremia, endotoxemia, and clinical correlates of sepsis [42].

Some of the causes of hemodynamic changes induced by CO_2 pneumoperitoneum are uncertain. Marathe demonstrated that despite significant and large increases in the arterial $PaCO_2$ beginning at intra-abdominal pressures of 5 mmHg, hemodynamic alterations only occurred when the $PaCO_2$ increased by 33%, and no change in mean arterial pressure was observed despite significant alterations in the arterial $PaCO_2$ and increased intra-abdominal pressure [44]. This discrepancy suggests that deleterious effects in hemodynamic and cardiovascular function needs two circumstances: long duration of CO_2 insufflation and high intra-abdominal pressure. To ameliorate the adverse effects of CO_2 pneumoperitoneum, some investigators have suggested the use of alternative gases or abdominal wall retraction devices [43].

Alternative Gases to Pneumoperitoneum

Nitrous Oxide

Diagnostic endoscopists even now prefer nitrous oxide as an alternative gas for diagnostic laparoscopy performed in patients under local anesthesia. Nitrous oxide produces less peritoneal irritation and less pain, allowing laparoscopy in the awake patient. Since electrocautery is not used under these circumstances, the risk of explosion is slight. If one would consider nitrous oxide as an alternative gas for operative laparoscopy it should be taken into account that nitrous oxide will diffuse into any closed gas space and will support combustion if present in a high enough concentration. The transfer rate of nitrous oxide into the peritoneal cavity, after the creation of a pneumoperitoneum with air, has been reported to be very rapid [5]. There are reports in the literature of abdominal explosion, even resulting in death [2, 3]. During laparoscopic surgery, if the nitrous oxide concentration in the peritoneal cavity reaches levels that could support combustion of highly volatile bowel gas (methane and hydrogen), an explosion hazard could exist. If a bowel perforation is recognized during laparoscopy, the peritoneal cavity should be vented and purged with carbon dioxide, and nitrous oxide removed from the anesthetic mixture [6]. This important problem led to the gradual renunciation of nitrous oxide as an insufflation agent in favor of carbon dioxide. Nitrous oxide is obviously not suitable if surgical intervention is needed, since electrocoagulation cannot be used. Though some surgeons still favor nitrous oxide for diagnostic laparoscopy, it is even possible to use room air and, in developing countries some surgeons insufflate using a hand-held sigmoidoscope balloon [7].

Helium

Insufflation with inert gases such as helium or argon has some potential advantages, including their lower solubility in water, which avoids problems associated with absorption from the peritoneal cavity and injured surfaces, and also prevents condensation on the optics. These "new" gases are still in an early stage of evaluation, and further experimental and clinical investigations are required to assess their efficiency, safety, and cost/benefit ratio [45]. Employing helium and argon could be a solution to the possible deleterious effects of carbon dioxide abdominal insufflation. Some authors have published their limited experience with helium in human beings, while knowledge about argon is, as yet, at an experimental stage [35, 46, 47].

It has been suggested that helium is more appropriate than carbon dioxide since it is both inert and minimally absorbed, intra-abdominal pressure is increased without the introduction of an exogenous CO_2 load, and it causes less acidosis [32, 48]. Helium is, however, poorly soluble in blood, with a solubility coefficient of 0.00098 in human blood at 37°C. Helium appears not to be an ideal gas for pneumoperitoneum since it poses a much greater threat than carbon dioxide in the case of accidental gas embolism. Venous gas embolism with inert gases (argon, nitrogen, helium) has a significantly greater hemodynamic aftermath than with more soluble gases, such as nitrous oxide or carbon dioxide. Nevertheless, helium is more diffusible than CO_2 because of its low density; this may aid in the dissolution of small helium emboli in the blood to a degree approaching that of CO_2 [49, 50]. Khan et al. demonstrated that emboli of air, pure nitrogen, or pure oxygen cause bronchoconstriction, while on the contrary emboli of CO_2 or helium do not [51]. Helium emboli may, therefore, behave in a similar manner to CO_2 emboli because of rapid diffusibility and minimal effect on pulmonary mechanics [49]. In an experimental study animals that were embolized with inert gases (such as argon, nitrogen, or helium) rapidly developed respiratory and metabolic acidosis with the death of all animals. However, when the gas used was soluble (such as nitrous oxide or carbon dioxide) animals did not have relevant cardiovascular and hemodynamic changes [52]. Table 2 shows the characteristics of different gases used in laparoscopy.

To maintain the established benefits of minimal access surgery in high-risk patients, some authors have suggested the use of helium for insufflation. The absence of the hypercarbia, acidemia, and pulmonary hypertension that characterize carbon dioxide pneumoperitoneum suggests that helium may be the insufflating agent of choice in patients with significant cardiopulmonary diseases. However, hemodynamic studies observed changes in relation to inferior vena cava pressure (IVCP) and portal vein pressure (PVP) to be increased in both groups, helium and CO_2, due to high intraperitoneal pressure [56]. The mean

Table 2. Characteristics of different pneumoperitoneum gases

	Carbon dioxide	Nitrous oxide	Air	Argon	Helium	Oxygen
Inert	–	+	+	+	+	–
Combustible	–	+	+	–	–	+
Water soluble	+	–	–	–	–	–
Peritoneal irritation (abdominal pain)	+	–	+	–	–	+

+, yes; -, no.

arterial pressures (MAP), mean pulmonary arterial pressures (MPAP), and mean pulmonary arterial wedge pressures (MPAWP) exhibited minimal but statistical changes in Leighton's study [2], in contrast to Shuto's observation [53] of no significant differences between the two groups.

Results comparing the cardiac output (CO) of the two gases remain controversial. The most valuable changes in CO are in relation to intra-abdominal pressure independent of the type of gas. [14, 17, 49, 53, 54]. Shuto did not find differences between the helium and CO_2 groups with a decreased blood flow associated with increased intra-abdominal pressure [53].

Blood gas analyses show that $PaCO_2$ increased significantly in CO_2 pneumoperitoneum compared with the helium insufflation group [35, 48, 53]. Analyses of pH levels were slightly lower in the CO_2 group. However, hydrocarbonate ion (HCO_3^-) was similar in both groups. In our observations comparing hemodynamic and blood gas changes in prolonged CO_2 versus helium pneumoperitoneum (see Table 3), we obtained results similar to those of other studies. Changes in delivery of O_2 (DO_2), consumption of O_2 (VO_2), and extraction ratio (ER) of oxygen as a result of a long-lasting pneumoperitoneum reflect the fact that CO_2 insufflation has a more harmful effect on systemic tissue oxygen uptake than helium pneumoperitoneum [55].

In further clinical studies performed by our group comparing laparoscopic cholecystectomy with carbon dioxide and helium pneumoperitoneum, insufflation with helium did not result in an increase in ventilation requirement although, as with CO_2 pneumoperitoneum, it was associated with a mean rise in peak airway pressure. CO_2 insufflation significantly increased $PaCO_2$; however, CO_2 and helium pneumoperitoneum each resulted in metabolic acidosis. The decreased pH levels were explained by respiratory acidosis in patients with significant $PaCO_2$ level increases [57]. Moreover, several studies suggest that acidosis was due to impairment of tissue perfusion, decreased CO with lactic acidosis, and impairment of regional oxygenation/perfusion [41, 53, 58]. The impairment of tissue perfusion and subsequent metabolic acidosis in relation to prolonged intraperitoneal pressure has more hemodynamic consequence than the self-same hypercarbia demonstrated in patients during carbon dioxide insufflation [41, 53, 59, 60].

Although more clinical studies with alternative gases should be undertaken, we have learned that helium pneumoperitoneum is not associated with significant hypercarbia, respiratory acidosis, or increased pulmonary artery pressure.

Table 3. Hemodynamic and gasometric effects of experimental laparoscopy in 12 pigs with CO_2 pneumoperitoneum and heliumpneumoperitoneum at 15 mmHg of intra-abdominal pressure maintained during 90 min (T1). To is baseline.

	CO_2pneumoperitoneum		Heliumpneumoperitoneum	
	T0	T1	T0	T1
HR (beat/min)	105 ± 22	108 ± 28	105 ± 27	95 ± 26
CO (l/min)	2.6 ± 1	1.6 ± 0.7*	2.1 ± 0.5	1.3 ± 0.1*
MAP (mmHG)	85 ± 28	84 ± 22	76 ± 20	78 ± 20
MPAP (mmHG)	24 ± 3	32 ± 6	25 ± 3	28 ± 5
PWP (mmHG)	10 ± 2	14 ± 2*	11 ± 2	14 ± 2*
FVP (mmHG)	10 ± 4	22 ± 1*	9 ± 2	22 ± 3*
HBF (ml/min)	452 ± 222	301 ± 115 **	464 ± 182	195 ± 79**
pHa	7.46 ± 0.05	7.31 ± 0.07**	7.45 ± 0.10	7.38 ± 0.09**
pHv	7.42 ± 0.06	7.24 ± 0.09**	7.39 ± 0.09	7.32 ± 0.10**
pHsh	7.41 ± 0.08	7.22 ± 0.03*	7.42 ± 0.06	7.24 ± 0.09*
pCO_2a (mmHG)	31 ± 8	49 ± 11 (+58%)**	33 ± 10	40 ± 13 (21%)**
pCO_2v (mmHG)	33 ± 7	61 ± 14 (85%)**	41 ± 11	53 ± 17 (+29%)**
pCO_2sh (mmHG)	33 ± 3	69 ± 15 (+109%)**	46 ± 10	63 ± 16 (+37%)**
CaO_2 (ml/dl)	13.2 ± 1.2	13.3 ± 1.1	13.8 ± 1.7	14.3 ± 1.8
CvO_2 (ml/dl)	10.6 ± 1.3	9.7 ± 1.8	11.2 ± 2.2	9.9 ± 1.5
$CsgO_2$ (ml/dl)	7.1 ± 0.8	5.4 ± 1.1**	6.8 ± 0.6	4.3 ± 0.9**

HR, heart rate; CO, cardiac output; MAP, mean arterial blood pressure; MPAP, mean pulmonary arterial pressure; PWP, pulmonary wedge pressure; FVP, femoral venous pressure; HBF, hepatic blood flow; a, arterial; v, mixed venous; sh, suprahepatic vein.

* $p < 0.05$ with respect to T0
** $p < 0.05$ with respect to T0 and $p < 0.05$ between groups

The pulmonary hypertension and the elevation in pulmonary vascular resistance that are observed during CO_2 but not helium insufflation are primarily due to the increased CO_2 content and decreased pH of the venous blood and not to hypoxic vasoconstriction. However, the low water solubility of helium obliges us to utilize some maneuvers to prevent possible gas embolism such as initiating pneumoperitoneum with open Hasson's technique or with CO_2 through the Veress needle, changing afterward to helium insufflation.

In our institute, helium pneumoperitoneum is used in patients with pheocromocytoma. There are still no comparative studies with a CO_2 group; however, it is well-known that CO_2 stimulates the sympathetic nervous system. In a comparative clinical study in patients with pheocromocytoma undergoing adrenalectomy by either open surgery or the laparoscopic approach, Fernandez-Cruz found a markedly greater increase in plasma norepinephrine and epinephrine in the open group. It is possible to relate these changes in plasma catecholamine concentrations to tumor manipulation; however, in the laparoscopic group they did not find any correlation between elevated catecholamine levels and hemodymamic and cardiovascular changes [61]. More investigations comparing the "new gases" with carbon dioxide and their effects on catecholamine response and organ blood flow changes are needed.

Carbon Dioxide, Alternative Gases, and Malignancy

Another important reason for finding alternative methods of exposure for minimally invasive surgery is that some animal studies suggest that insufflation of the peritoneal cavity with carbon dioxide is a potential causative factor in the development of abdominal wall metastases after resection of malignant tumors. Some experimental studies have been performed in animal models to study peritoneal growth and abdominal wall metastases after carbon dioxide and air pneumoperitoneum, gasless laparoscopy, and laparotomy. Carbon dioxide could also act as a vehiculum for tumor cells, transporting cells from the tumor to sites susceptible to tumor take due to ischemia [62]. The results in the literature are controversial. In a paper published recently, Hubens et al. [63] conclude that the presence of a pneumoperitoneum does not enhance the implantation of free malignant colon cancer cells in rats. In a different experimental study, it has been reported that insufflation of carbon dioxide promotes tumor growth compared to the control group in a rat model. Use of carbon dioxide appears to stimulate tumor growth [64]; however, Jacobi suggests that helium does not stimulate cell growth in vitro and in vivo [65]. In summary, the use of helium to create pneumoperitoneum may provide a safer alternative for abdominal insufflation, especially in patients with pre-existing cardiac and/or pulmonary dysfunction, malignant diseases, or patients with anomalous catecholamine secretion such as pheocromocytoma. Nevertheless, we do not recommend the utilization of helium in healthy patients and patients with severe liver or renal dysfunction.

Conclusions

We are confident that alternative gases will take their place in the creation of pneumoperitoneum and contribute to the well-documented benefits of laparoscopic surgery. Further controlled trials are necessary to determine the benefits and risks of pneumoperitoneum performed with differing gases.

References

1. Fervers C (1933) Die Laparoskopie mit dem Cystokop. Med Klin 29:1042–1045
2. Edgerton W (1974) Laparoscopy in the community hospital: setup, performance, control. In: Phillips J, Keith L (eds) Gynecological laparoscopy: principles and techniques. Straton Intercontinental, New York, pp 79–90

3. El-Kady A, Abd-El-Razek M (1976) Intraperitoneal explosion during female sterilization by laparoscopic electrocoagulation. Int J Gynaecol Obstet 14:487–488

4. Gunatilake D(1978) Fatal intraperitoneal explosion during electrocoagulation via laparoscopy. Int J Gynaecol Obstet 15:353–357

5. Johnson W (1971) Pneumoeperitoneum for ventral hernia repair: anesthesia complications. JAMA 271:968

6. Neuman GG, Sidebotham G, Negoianu E, Bernstein J, Kopman AF, Hicks RG, West ST, Haring L (1993) Laparoscopy explosion hazards with nitrous oxide. Anesthesiology 78:875–879

7. Udwadia T (1986) Peritoneoscopy for surgeons. Ann R Coll Surg Engl 68:125–129

8. Kleinhaus S, Sammartano R, Boley S (1978) Effects of laparoscopy on mesenteric blood flow. Arch Surg 113:867–869

9. Melville R, Frizis H, Forsling M, LeQuesne L (1985) The stimulus for vasopressin release during laparoscopy. Surg Gynecol Obstet 161:253–256

10. Witten C, Andrus C, Fitzgerald S, Baudendistel L, Dahms T, Karminski D (1991) Analysis of hemodynamic and ventilatory effects of laparoscopic cholecystectomy. Arch Surg 126:997–1001

11. Myles P (1991) Bradyarrhythmias and laparoscopy: a prospective study of heart rate changes with laparoscopy. Aust N Z J Obstet Gynaecol 31:171–173

12. Liu S, Leighton T, Davis I, Klein S, Lippmann M, Bongard F (1991) Prospective analysis of cardiopulmonary responses to laparoscopic cholecystectomy. J Laparoendosc Surg 5:241–246

13. Westerband A, Van De Water J, Amzallag M, Lebowitz P, Nwasokwa O, Chardavoyne R, Abou-Taleb A, Wang X, Wise L (1992) Cardiovascular changes during laparoscopic cholecystectomy. Surg Gynecol Obstet 175:535–538

14. Ho H, Gunther R, Wolfe B (1992) Intraperitoneal carbon dioxide insufflation and cardiopulmonary functions. Arch Surg 127:928–933

15. Diebel L, Dulchavsky S, Wilson R (1992) Effect of increased intra-abdominal pressure on mesenteric arterial and intestinal mucosal blood flow. J Trauma 33:45–49

16. Volz J, Koster S, Weis M, Schmidt R, Urbaschek R, Melchert F, Albrecht M (1996) Pathophysiology features of a pneumoperitoneum at laparoscopy: a swine model. Am J Obstet Gynecol 174:132–140

17. Marshall R, Jebson P, Davie I, Scott D (1972) Circulatory effects of carbon dioxide insufflation of the peritoneal cavity for laparoscopy. Br J Anaesth 44:680–684

18. Barnett R, Gordon S, Drizin G (1992) Pulmonary changes after laparoscopic cholecystectomy. Surg Laprosc Endosc 2:125–127

19. Fitzgerald S, Andrus C, Baudendistel L, Dahms T, Kaminski D (1992) Hypercarbia during carbon dioxide pneumoperitoneum. Am J Surg 163:186–190

20. Kasten J, Green J, Parson E, Holeroft J (1981) Hemodynamic effects of increased abdominal pressure. J Surg Res 30:249–255

21. Ho H, Saunders C, Corso F (1993) The effect of CO_2 pneumoperitoneum on hemodynamics in hemorrhaged animals. Surgery 114:381–388

22. Kelman G, Swapp G, Smith I, Benzie R, Gordon N (1972) Cardiac output and arterial blood-gas tension during laparoscopy. Br J Anaesth 44:1155–1161

23. Lenz R, Thomas T, Wilkins D (1976) Cardiovascular changes during laparoscopy. Anaesthesia 31:4–12

24. Luiz T, Huber T, Hartung H (1992) Veränderungen der Ventilation während laparoskopischer Cholezystektomie. Anaesthesist 41:520–526

25. Moffa R, Quinn J, Slotman G (1993) Hemodynamic effects of carbon dioxide pneumoperitoneum during mechanical ventilation and positive end-expiratory pressure. J Trauma 35:613–617

26. Moten M, Ivankovich A, Bieniarz J, Albrecht R, Zahed B, Scommegna A (1973) Cardiovascular effects and acid-base and blood gas changes during laparoscopy. Am J Obstet Gynecol 115:1002–1012

27. Tolksdorf W, Strang C, Schippers E, Simon H, Truong S (1992) The effects of the carbon dioxide pneumoperitoneum in laparoscopic cholecystectomy on postoperative spontaneous respiration. Anesthesiology 41:199–203

28. Diamant M, Benumof J, Saidman L (1978) Hemodynamics of increased intraabdominal pressure: interaction with hypovolemia and halothane anesthesia. Anesthesiology 48:23–27

29. Ishizaki Y, Bandai Y, Kazuyuki S, Abe H, Ohtomo Y, Idezuke Y (1993) Safe intraabdominal pressure of carbon dioxide pneumoperitoneum during laparoscopic surgery. Surgery 114:549–554

30. Ishizaki Y, Bandai Y, Shimomura K, Abe H, Ohtomo Y, ldezuke Y (1993) Changes in splanchnic blood flow and cardiovascular effects following peritoneal insufflation of carbon dioxide. Surg Endosc 7:420–423
31. Johannsen G, Andersen M, Juhl B (1989) The effect of general anesthesia on the hemodynamic events during laparoscopy with CO_2 insufflation. Acta Anaesthesiol Scand 33:132–136
32. Leighton T, Pianim N, Liu SY, Kono M, Klein S, Bongard F (1992) Effects of hypercarbia during experimental pneumoperitoneum. Am Surg 58:717–721
33. Rasmussen J, Dauchot P, DePalma R (1978) Cardiac function and hypercarbia. Arch Surg 113:1196–1200
34. Safran D, Orlando R (1994) Physiologic effects of pneumoepritoneum. Am J Surg 167:281–286
35. Ivankovich A, Miletich D, Albrecht R, Heyman H, Bonnet R (1975) Cardiovascular effects of intraperitoneal insufflation with carbon dioxide and nitrous oxide in the dog. Anesthesiology 42:281–287
36. Alexander G, Brown E (1969) Physiologic alterations during pelvic laparoscopy. Am J Obstet Gynecol 105:1078–1081
37. Brown D, Fishburne J, Roberson V, Hulka J (1976) Ventilatory and blood gas changes during laparoscopy with local anesthesia. Am J Obstet Gynecol 124:741–745
38. Seed R, Shakespeare T, Muldoon M (1970) Carbon dioxide homeostasis during anesthesia for laparoscopy. Anaesthesia 25:223–231
39. Calweli C, Ricotta J (1987) Changes in visceral blood flow with elevated intraabdominal pressure. J Surg Res 43:14–20
40. Luca A, Cirera I, Garcia-Pagan J, Feu F, Pizcueta P, Bosch J, Rodes J (1993) Hemodynamic effects of acute changes in intra-abdominal pressure in patients with cirrhosis. Gastroenterology 104:222–227
41. Taurd P, Lopez A, Lacy AM, Anglada T, Beltran J, Fernandez-Cruz L, Targarona EM, Garcia-Vaidecasas JC, Merin JL (in press) Is the high pressure of pneumoperitoneum the cause of lactic acidosis? Surg Endosc
42. Gurtner G, Robertson C, Chung S, Ling T, Ip S, Li A (1995) Effects of carbon dioxide pneumoperitoneum on bacteraemia and endotoxaemia in an animal model of peritonitis. Br J Surg 82:844–848
43. Davidson B, Cromeens D, Feig B (1996) Alternative methods of exposure minimize cardiopulmonary risk in experimental animals during minimally invasive surgery. Surg Endosc 10:301–304
44. Maratha U, Lilly R, Silvestry S, Schauer PR, Davis JW, Pappas TN, Gower DD (1996) Alterations in hemodynamics and left ventricular contractility during carbon dioxide pneumoperitoneum. Surg Endosc 10:974–978
45. Berci G (1995) Pneumoperitoneum. In: Phillips E, Rosenthal R (eds) Operative strategies in laparoscopic surgery. Springer, Berlin Heidelberg New York, pp 13–18
46. Rademaker B, Odoom J, de Wit L, Kaikman C, ten Brink S, Ringers J (1994) Haemodynamic effects of pneumoperitoneum for laparoscopic surgery: a comparison of CO_2 with N_{20} insufflation. Eur J Anaesthesiol 11:301–306
47. Eisenhauer D, Saunders C, Ho H, Wolfe B (1994). Hemodynamic effects of argon pneumoperitoneum. Surg Endosc 8:315–321
48. Leighton T, Bongard F, Liu S-Y, Lee T, Klein S (1991) Comparative cardiopulmonary effects of helium and carbon dioxide pneumoperitoneum. Surg Forum 42:485–487
49. Leighton T, Liu S-Y, Bongard F (1993) Comparative cardiopulmonary effects of carbon dioxide versus helium pneumoperitoneum. Surgery 113:527–531
50. Bongard F, Pianim N, Leighton T, Dubecz S, Davis IP, Lippmann M, Klein S, Liu SY (1993) Helium insufflation for laparoscopic operation. Surg Gynecol Obstet 177:140–146
51. Khan M, Alkalay I, Suetsugu S, Stein M (1972) Acute changes in lung mechanics following pulmonary emboli of various gases in dogs. J Appl Physiol 33:774–777
52. Roberts M, Mathiesen K, Wolfe B (1995) Venous gas embolization model for laparoscopic surgery. Surg Endosc 9:A210 (abstr)
53. Shuto K, Kitano S, Yoshida T, Bandoh T, Mitarai Y, Kobayashi M (1995) Hemodynamic and arterial blood changes during carbon dioxide and helium pneumoperitoneum in pigs. Surg Endosc 9:1173–1179
54. Motew M, Ivankovich A, Bieniarz J, Albrecht RF, Zahed B, Scommegna A, Silverman B (1973) Cardiovascular effects and acid-base and blood changes during laparoscopy. Am J Obstet Gynecol 115:1002–1012

55. Martinez-Palif G, Delgado S, Fontanals J, Lacy AM, Pacheco JL, Taura P, Visa J (1996) Hemodynamic changes during prolonged pneumoperitoneum with carbon dioxide or helium. Surg Endosc 10:245 (abstr)
56. Sala Blanch X, Fontanals J, Delgado S, Martinez-Palif G, Taura P, Lacy AM, Visa J (1996) Effects of carbon dioxide versus helium pneumoperitoneum on hepatic blood flow in pigs. Surg Endosc 10:183 (abstr)
57. McMahon A, Baxter J, Murray W, Imrie C, Kenny G, O'Dwyer P (1994) Helium pneumoperitoneum for laparoscopic cholecystectomy: ventilatory and blood gas changes. Br J Surg 81:1033–1036
58. Shenasky J, Gifiewater J (1972) The renal hemodynamic and functional effects of external counterpressure. Surg Gynecol Obstet 134:253–258
59. Cohen R, Woods H (1976) The clinical presentations and classifications of lactic acidosis. In: Cohen R, Woods H (eds) Clinical and biochemical aspects of lactic acidosis. Blackwell, Oxford, p 42
60. Hashikura Y, Kawasaki S, Munakata Y, Hashimoto S, Hayashi K, Makuuchi M (1994) Effects of peritoneal insufflation on hepatic and renal blood flow. Surg Endosc 18:759–761
61. Fernandez-Cruz L, Taura P, Saenz A, Benarroch G, Sabater L (1996) Laparoscopic approach to pheocromocytoma: hemodynamic changes and catecholamine secretion. World J Surg 20:762–768
62. Wu L, Mustoe T (1995) Effect of ischemia on growth factor enhancement of incisional wound healing. Surgery 117:570–576
63. Hubens G, Pauwels M, Hubens A, Vermeuien P, Van Merck E, Eyskens E (1996) The influence of a pneumoperitoneum on the peritoneal implantation of free intraperitoneal colon cancer cells. Surg Endosc 10:809–812
64. Bouvy N, Marquet R, Hamming J, Jeekel J, Bonjer H (1996) Laparoscopic surgery in the rat. Beneficial effect on body weight and tumor take. Surg Endosc 10:490–494
65. Jacobi C, Sabat R, Bohm B, Zieren H, Volk H, Muller J (1996) Pneumoperitoneum with CO_2 stimulates malignant tumor growth. Surg Endosc 551 (abstr)

3 Influence of Gas Temperature During Laparoscopic Procedures

J.R. Bessell and G.J. Maddern

Introduction

Therapeutic laparoscopy has been rapidly accepted worldwide and currently accounts for an increasing proportion of intra-abdominal procedures, yet the influence of laparoscopic surgery on perioperative temperature homeostasis has received little attention. Evidence is emerging to suggest that the nature of insuflated gas plays a substantial role in the development or prevention of hypothermia during laparoscopy.

Before considering the impact of insufflated gas, it is important to understand the pathogenesis and effects of perioperative hypothermia. Hypothermia has been defined as core temperature below 36° C [14] and results from the influence of anesthesia, augmented by certain characteristics of the individual patient.

Influence of General Anesthesia

General anesthesia influences the development of intraoperative hypothermia by disturbing thermal regulatory mechanisms. This occurs in three phases [22]:

1. In the first instance, anesthesia reduces the thermoregulatory threshold for vasoconstriction by 2.5 C, resulting in a core-to-peripheral redistribution of body heat [22].
2. A second decrease in body temperature is a result of heat loss exceeding metabolic heat production. Heat production decreases only minimally during anesthesia [26], and respiratory heat loss is relatively small [3], therefore, the predominant site of heat loss is cutaneous. For example, exposure of the unclad, immobile patient to the cool theatre environment [14–16], evaporative water losses from surgical incisions [14], evaporation of surgical skin preparation solution, and the use of cold intravenous infusions or irrigating fluids [9, 23] can all cause heat loss through the skin. Certain types of surgery, such as laparotomy, contribute to loss of heat from surgical incisions by increasing the surface area of the patient available for heat exchange [19, 27].
3. After 3–4 hours, core temperature finally reaches a plateau. Patients that are kept relatively warm require no active thermoregulation at this stage. If not kept warm, thermoregulatory vasoconstriction decreases cutaneous heat loss [21], and sequesters metabolic heat to the core [1].

Influence of Patient Characteristics

Patient characteristics such as age, size, and associated medical conditions augment both the degree of hypothermia and also the resultant effects. For example, in elderly patients with limited cardiopulmonary reserves, marked postoperative thermogenic shivering can dramatically increase oxygen consumption, risking cardiac arrythmias, failure, or myocardial infarction [8, 27].

Effects of Perioperative Hypothermia

The importance of perioperative hypothermia becomes apparent when the numerous deleterious effects it may cause are considered. Conditions such as increased susceptibility to dermal infection [24], induction of a hypokalemic state [4, 11], impaired myocardial function [12], respiratory depression, negative nitrogen balance [5], thrombocytopenia, and depletion of clotting factors [7] have been reported.

The net effect of these complications is reflected in the mortality rate of patients thus affected. One study reported a 24% mortality in postoperative patients who remained hypothermic for 2 hours, compared with 4% of their normothermic counterparts [25]. There is a financial penalty as well since hypothermic patients are reported to spend up to 1 hours longer in the recovery ward [6], and a mean increase in length of hospital stay of 2.6 days was recently demonstrated for patients with postoperative temperatures less than 35.5°C [10].

Impact of Laparoscopy on Perioperative Hypothermia

Until recently it had been assumed that the impact of laparoscopy would be to decrease the risk of heat loss by comparison with the corresponding "open" procedure. This assumption was based on the knowledge that the predominant thermal loss during surgery is from exposed surfaces. During laparotomy the open abdomen exposes a greater surface area, whereas during laparoscopy with the abdomen sealed there was believed to be less potential heat loss from convection, as well as conduction, and radiation. Yet the abdomen is not sealed off from the environment during laparoscopy. Indeed, gas flow rates passing over peritoneal surfaces during insufflation may exceed those during open laparotomy.

Furthermore, laparoscopic procedures may take longer to perform than their open counterparts, predisposing the patient to greater heat losses from prolonged exposure in the anesthetized state.

Experimental and clinical data now indicate that during laparoscopy heat loss also occurs due to the use of CO_2 gas which is insufflated into the peritoneal cavity to provide surgical access. Laparoscopic insufflators use high-pressure bottles as the source of CO_2. In delivering gas from a bottle source to the patient, the gas pressure must be brought from a pressure in the range 1350 mmHg (180 kPa) to 37|600 mmHg (5000 kPa) down to a pressure of 15 mmHg (2 kPa). Associated with the change of pressure at the regulator is gas expansion. As the gas expands, it cools, and as it is in contact with the regulator, this also cools. The degree of cooling is dependent on the flow rate; at high gas-flow rates the cooling will be more pronounced.

Some laparoscopic procedures require only modest CO_2 flow rates; however, other advanced laparoscopic procedures such as colorectal and esophageal operations frequently result in large gas leaks due to the use of multiple large ports of up to 33 mm in diameter, insertion and removal of laparoscopic instruments, extraction of electrocautery smoke which may obscure vision, aspiration of gas by the sucker as intraperitoneal fluid is removed, and inadvertent removal of ports not fixed securely to the abdominal wall. Insufflation may therefore be required at high flow rates to maintain adequate pneumoperitoneum over a sustained period.

Because of the large numbers of patients undergoing laparoscopy, the uncorrected physiological insult of hypothermia, particularly during prolonged surgery, is considered to be a problem of considerable magnitude.

Experimental Data

At the Queen Elizabeth Hospital, South Australia, we have conducted two randomized crossover animal trials under controlled conditions to investigate the problem of laparoscopy-induced hypothermia. Ethical approval for both projects was granted by the animal ethics committees of The Queen Elizabeth Hospital and the University of Adelaide.

Methodology

The methodology was similar in both studies, utilizing six pigs of approximately 30 kg. In both studies, each animal received three different treatments on three separate occasions. The order of these treatments was randomized and performed 1 week apart.

In the first study, the three treatments involved insufflating the animal with cold dry gas (25°C, 2% relative humidity, RH) on one occasion, insufflating heated dry gas (30°C, 2% RH) on another occasion, and on an additional occasion, as a control procedure, no insufflation was performed. In the second study, the three treatments involved insufflating the animal with cold dry gas (21°C, 2% RH) on one occasion, insufflating heated humidified gas (40°C, 98% RH) on another occasion, and as a control procedure no insufflation was performed on an additional occasion. The pneumoperitoneal pressure was maintained at 10 mmHg. Insufflation was performed at 10 l/min by creating a standardized "leak" from a second supra-umbilical port. This was performed to simulate the repeated gas losses that are experienced clinically during some advanced laparoscopic operations.

Each pig was anesthetized and wrapped with a silver radiation blanket to reduce cutaneous heat loss, and was ventilated with a humidified circuit to reduce respiratory heat loss. The crossover design of this controlled methodology allowed us examine only laparoscopy-induced temperature changes, as heat loss to the environment and anesthetic circuit were standardized.

Core temperature was measured every 15 min by an esophageal thermoresistor, while ambient room temperature was maintained at a thermo-neutral 24°C. The observed core temperature changes for each of the three treatment groups in both studies were expressed as regression lines using repeated measures analysis of variance (RMANOVA). These lines, therefore, represent the temperature effect over time for all animals in the relevant treatment group.

Effect of Cold and Warm Insufflated CO_2

It was found that the regression lines summarizing changes over time for the cold dry gas and warmed dry gas treatment groups were statistically indistinguishable. Consequently, there was no significant temperature difference between animals that received cold dry gas or warmed dry gas over a 3-hour period, and these two groups can be considered to behave as one. The core temperature at the commencement of anesthesia for control animals that received no gas insufflation was 36.9°C; however, after 3 hours a significant rise to 37.2°C was recorded. The temperature at the commencement of anesthesia for animals that had cold dry or warmed dry gas insufflated was again 36.9°C, but fell to 36.1°C at 3 hours, a statistically significant difference of 0.8°C ($p < 0.001$). There was also a significant difference between the temperatures recorded by control animals and those undergoing gas insufflation ($p < 0.001$), a variation of 1.17°C after 3 hours (Fig. 1).

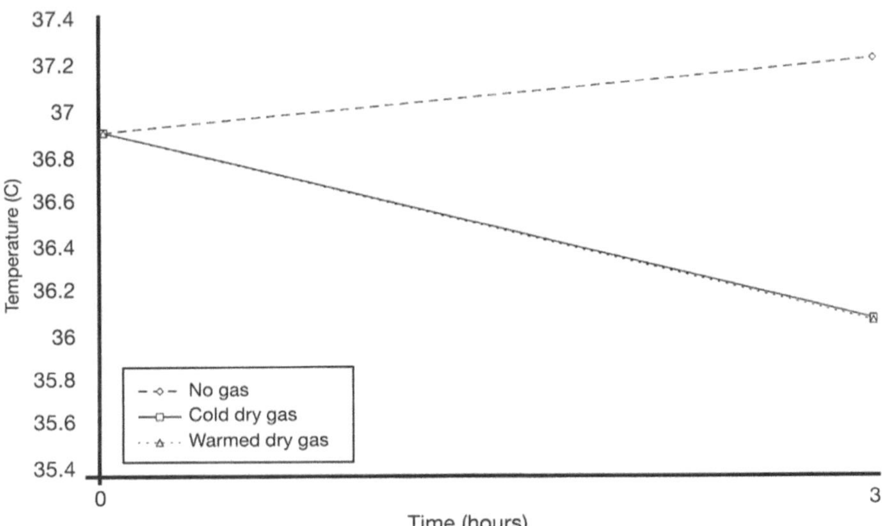

Fig. 1. Esophageal temperature in the study investigating the effect of cold and warm insufflated CO_2. Regression lines for cold and warmed dry gas were indistinguishable.

This was the first study to rigorously confirm that insufflation of CO_2 gas at high flow rates over a prolonged period of time results in a significant fall in core temperature [2]. The magnitude of this hypothermic effect due solely to laparoscopy would exert a clinically significant impact, especially when added to the numerous other factors tending to reduce body temperature during general anesthesia.

Although an average leak of 10 l/min is unlikely to be tolerated for prolonged periods in most laparoscopic operations, this exaggerated "worst-case" scenario was chosen as the model to unmask any effect which may be potentially disguised by a more clinically modest situation. It is also perhaps trivial that the difference between the cold and warmed gas was only 5°C, but this represented the limit of the capabilities of commercially available insufflators at the time of the study.

The second important fact emanating from this study was that provision of warmed rather than cold insufflated gas confers no protection against changes in core temperature during laparoscopic surgery. This has commercial implications since insufflators with built-in heating elements are marketed by some companies. Why was warmed gas no better, although it exited the insufflator 5° warmer than the cold gas? The answer is provided by the principles of thermodynamics; considerably more heat expenditure from the patient is required to humidify the initially dry CO_2 stream, than is used to raise the ambient temperature of the CO_2 gas to a physiological temperature.

A simple thermodynamic calculation indicates that the heat required to raise the temperature of the CO_2 gas flowing at 10 l/min from 25° to 37°C is 0.9 W, and the heat required to raise the temperature of the CO_2 gas from 30° to 37°C is 0.48 W. Both of these are minuscule in comparison to the basal metabolic rate of 80 W, and would reduce body temperature by less than 0.1°C over 3 hours. A further thermodynamic calculation shows that the latent heat required to evaporate body water in the pig to saturate the initially dry CO_2 stream of 10 l/min at 37°C is 18 W. This indicates that the evaporation of body water to saturate the CO_2 is a much greater source of heat requirement.

The third important fact emanating from this study was the suggestion that humidification of the insulated CO_2 would largely resolve the problem of laparoscopy-induced hypothermia. A second study, therefore, became inevitable to confirm the contribution of water evaporation to heat loss, and evaluate the efficacy of insulation with heated humidified gas in its prevention.

Effect of Humidifying Insufflated CO_2

When warmed humidified gas was substituted for warmed dry gas in the second study, the regression line summarizing changes over time was observed to be no longer superimposed on the results of the cold dry gas group, but moved up to become statistically indistinguishable from the "no gas" group (Fig. 2). This means that core temperatures after laparoscopic insulation with warmed humidified gas were no different to insufflated control animals. This is all the more remarkable considering the deliberately exaggerated gas losses of 10 l/min.

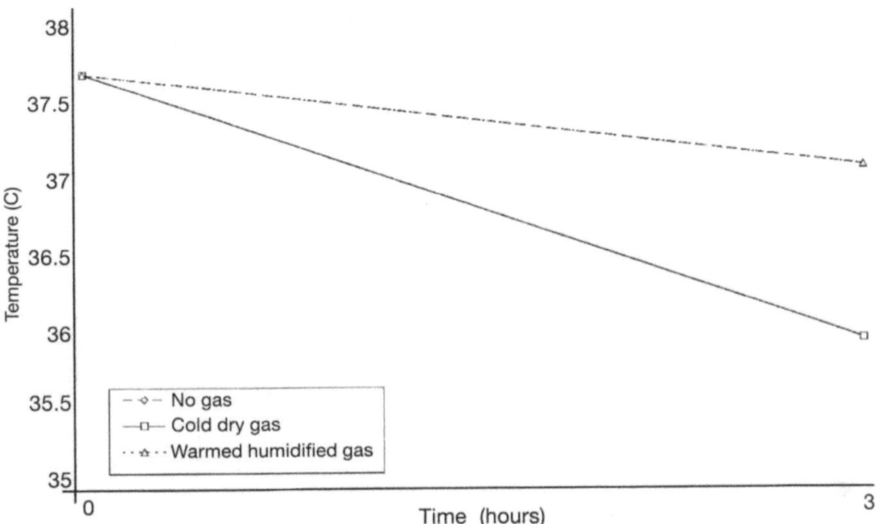

Fig. 2. Esophageal temperature in the study investigating the effect of humidifying insufflated CO_2. Regression line of warmed humidified gas and no gas are indistinguishable.

As before, after 3 hours of insulation with cold dry gas, core temperature fell significantly (by 1.77°C in this study). The temperature differential between the two lines (1.17°C), therefore, represents the energy that was lost by the animal heating and humidifying cold dry gas to physiological levels.

By measuring the temperature and relative humidity of gas entering and exiting the animal model, it was possible to thermodynamically calculate the predicted core temperature fall following insulation of an animal of 30 kg with cold dry gas. In these energy calculations, the component attributable to heating the insufflated CO_2 to physiological levels was ignored because of the extremely low specific heat of gas. Table 1 shows the values recorded by the sensors positioned to instantaneously measure the temperature and relative humidity of insulated and exsufflated gas. The predicted temperature drop due to water

Table 1. Temperature and relative humidity of insufflated and exsufflated gas

	Insufflated gas		Exsufflated gas	
	Temperature (°C)	Relative humidity (%)	Temperature (°C)	Relative humidity (%)
Cold dry gas	23.9 (21.9 – 25.9)	2[a]	31.4 (31 – 31.8)	88.2 (87 – 89.5)
Warmed humidifed gas	40.7 (39.5 – 42)	98.3 [a]	34.5 (34 – 35)	89.4 (87.7 – 91.2)

Values are means with 95 % confidence intervals.
[a] Consistent values established during in vitro experiments.

evaporation was calculated at a flow rate of 10 l/min for 3 hours assuming that the specific heat capacity of pig tissue is 3.5 kJ/kg, assuming a latent heat of vaporization of 2.43 J/mg, and assuming a saturated water content at 23.9°C and 31.4°C of 21 mg/l and 33 mg/l, respectively. The results confirmed that a large proportion of the temperature drop after insufflation of cold dry gas is due to the latent heat required for evaporation of body water to saturate the dry CO_2 stream, rather than the heat required to raise the cold gas to body temperature. The calculated mean temperature drop due to water evaporation was 1.2°C, which compares with the 1.17°C observed temperature difference between control animals and those insufflated with cold dry gas.

The close correlation between the calculated and measured temperature changes in pigs treated with cold dry gas strongly supports the hypothesis that prevention of water loss is the most important factor for the prevention of laparoscopic hypothermia.

Clinical Data

Before 1995, the literature contained five uncontrolled studies addressing the issue of laparoscopic hypothermia. Two emanated from the Georgia Biomedical Research Group, and were the most often cited. The first reported that changes in core temperature as a result of laparoscopy can be expected to drop by 0.3°C for each 50 l of CO_2 delivered [17]. The second study by the same group reported that postoperative temperatures in 20 patients receiving warmed CO_2 (35°– 35.5°C) were within 0.1°C of pre- and intraoperative values [18]. This contrasted to a control group receiving unwarmed CO_2 (21°C) where a thermal loss of 0.3°C per 50 l of consumed CO_2 was reported. Unfortunately, this valuable study was not randomized and different operations were performed both between and within groups. Non-commercial warming devices were used, and similar but not identical flow rates and volumes of CO_2 were used. These methodological factors could have introduced errors and the conclusion that the use of physiologic temperature CO_2 helps diminish thermal loss remained to be proven.

Three other studies reported uncontrolled clinical observations of the development of hypothermia during laparoscopic procedures. Wallasvaara reported in 1992 that thermal loss is at least comparable during open and laparoscopic cholecystectomy [28]. A retrospective analysis published in 1993 measured patients' temperatures during laparoscopic cases ranging between 3 and 6 hours, and observed an average initial temperature of 36.1°C falling to an average of 33.3°C. A total of 4–6 hours of rewarming was required in the recovery room to return the patient to a normal temperature [20]. A third study conducted in Australia, investigated 21 consecutive patients undergoing laparoscopic cholecystectomy with cold CO_2 insufflation [13]. The patients' rectal temperatures were studied for durations of between 30 and 60 min. There was a statistically, but not clinically, significant fall in temperature over the course of the procedures (36.4 ± 0.46–36.2 ± 0.35°C), although the authors admit that rectal temperature monitoring is often inaccurate with slow response times, and the relatively short duration of the study would preclude significant temperature changes being observed. The authors concluded that it was appropriate to maximize heat conservation for longer laparoscopic procedures.

Conclusions

Disturbed temperature physiology such as has been demonstrated by the overwhelming majority of available literature will not be problematic or apparent in every laparoscopic operation. By far the majority of laparoscopic procedures performed in routine practice are of modest duration and incur minimal gas leakage. However, it is important for the clinician utilizing non-humidified insufflation equipment to be aware of this potential problem for several reasons:

1. Hypothermia should be anticipated if the laparoscopic procedure is planned to be or becomes prolonged, or incurs large gas losses. Examples of such procedures are complex gastrointestinal procedures such as laparoscopic esophageal, gastric, colonic, or pancreatic resections. Also, if other cooling influences are present during anesthesia the hypothermic effect of laparoscopy could exert a clinically significant impact.
2. Appropriate heat conservation prophylaxis should be instituted in both these circumstances.
3. There may be a temptation to submit to commercial pressure to purchase gas-warming insufflators when in fact their touted benefits have no physiological validity.
4. Surgeons may assume that the purchase of gas-warming insufflators will protect their patients from hypothermia, perhaps forsaking other precautionary measures.

On the basis of experimental data, the use of warmed but also humidified gas to maintain temperature homeostasis during laparoscopy must be advocated. Unfortunately, we are unaware of any commercial units that have achieved the certified standards of electrical safety and sterility required for clinical use.

Summary

The current state of knowledge concerning the physiology of temperature balance during laparoscopy can be enumerated as follows (Fig. 3):

1. Mechanisms of hypothermia during general anesthesia include heat redistribution, disturbance of thermoregulatory mechanisms, and use of cold intravenous infusions. A major component is heat loss from exposed surfaces, a situation accelerated by a cool theatre environment, evaporation of surgical skin preparation solution, exposed body cavities during surgery, or the use of cold irrigating fluids.
2. Patient characteristics such as age, size, and associated medical conditions augment both the degree of hypothermia and also the resultant effects.

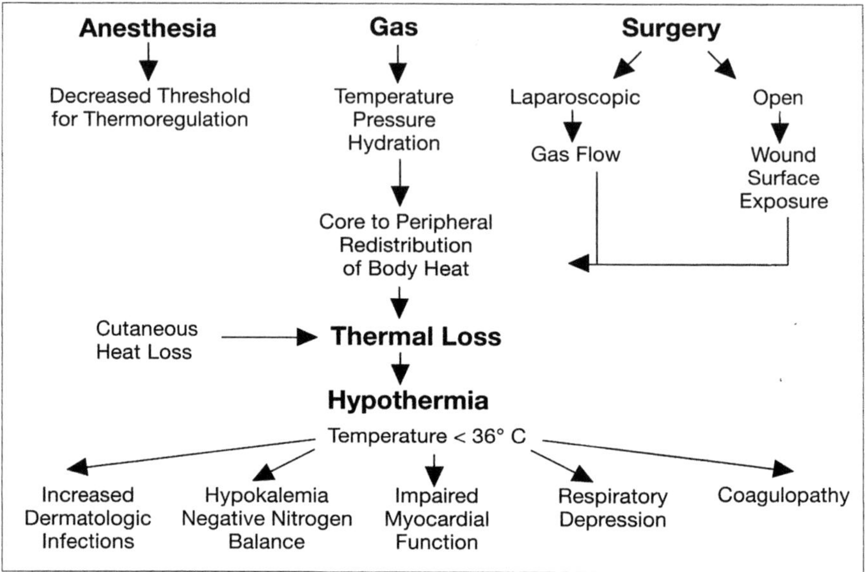

Fig. 3. Summary of the effects of gas temperature during laparoscopic procedures

3. Cool dry CO_2 at 21°C and 0% relative humidity is the standard gas that emanates from the patient outlet of the majority of unmodified commercially available insufflators. While some warming and humidification occurs during passage along insufflator tubing, this is minimal, and contributes little to heat conservation.

4. Controlled animal studies have confirmed that insufflation of the CO_2 gas supplied with standard laparoscopic units results in a significant fall in core body temperature, when used at high flow rates over a prolonged period of time.

5. Currently available insufflators with built-in heating elements for the warming of insufflated gas confer no protection against laparoscopy-induced hypothermia.

6. The intra-abdominal CO_2 during laparoscopic surgery is at body temperature and nearly 100% saturated with body water.

7. The theoretical principles of thermodynamics indicate that considerably more heat expenditure from the patient would be needed to evaporate body water to humidify the initially dry CO_2 stream, than would be required to raise the ambient temperature of the CO_2 gas to body temperature.

There is experimental data from controlled animal studies confirming the theory that vaporization of water is a major component of heat loss during laparoscopy, and that humidification of insuflated CO_2 can minimize the problem of laparoscopy-induced hypothermia.

References

1. Belani KG, Sessler DI, Larson NM et al (1993) The pupillary light reflex: effects of anesthetics and hyperthermia. Anesthesiology 79:23–27
2. Bessell JR, Karatassas A, Jamieson GG, Maddem GJ. (1995) Hypothermia induced by laparoscopic insulation: a randomized study in a pig model. Surg Endosc 9:791–795
3. Bickler P, Sessler DI. (1990) Efficiency of airway heat and moisture exchangers in anesthetized humans. Anesth Analg 71:415–418
4. Boelhouwer R, Bruining H, Ong G (1987) Correlations of serum potassium fluctuations with body temperature after major surgery. Crit Care Med 15:310–312
5. Carli F, Emery PW, Freemantle CAJ (1989) Effect of perioperative normothermia on postoperative protein metabolism in elderly patients undergoing hip arthroplasty. Br J Anaesth 63:276–282
6. Conahan TJ. (1982) Heating reduces recovery time (cost) in outpatients. Anesthesiology 67:128–130
7. Ellis P, Kleinsaser L, Speer R (1957) Changes in coagulation occurring in dogs during hypothermia and cardiac surgery. Surgery 41:198–210
8. Heymann AD (1977) The effect of incidental hypothermia on elderly surgical patients. J Gerontol 32:146–148
9. Imrie MM, Hall GM (1991) Body temperature and anaesthesia. Br J Anaesth 64:346354
10. Kurz A, Sessler DI, Lenhardt R (1996) Perioperative normothermia to reduce the incidence of surgical wound infection and shorten hospitalization. N Engl J Med 334:1209–1215
11. Laszlo A, Sprung J, Polic S, Kampine JP, Bosnjak ZJ (1990) Effects of hypothermia and potassium variations on maximum diastolic potential. Anesthesiology 73:3A
12. Mattheussen A, Boutros A, Van Aken H, Flameng W (1990) Effect of the volatile anesthetics on the hypothermic myocardium. Anesthesiology 73:A574
13. Monagle J, Bradfield S, Nottle P (1993) Carbon dioxide, temperature and laparoscopic cholecystectomy. Aust N Z J Surg 63:186–189
14. Morris RH, Ktunar A (1972) The effect of warming blankets on maintenance of body temperature of the anesthetized, paralyzed adult patient. Anesthesiology 36:408–411
15. Morris RH, Wilkey B (1970) The effects of ambient temperature on patient temperature during surgery not involving body cavities. Anesthesiology 32:102–107
16. Morris RH (1971) Influence of ambient temperature on patient temperature during intraabdominal surgery. Ann Surg 173(2):230–233
17. Ott DE(1991a) Laparoscopic hypothermia. J Laparoendosc Surg 1:127–31
18. Oft DE (1991b) Correction of laparoscopic insulation hypothermia. J Laparoendosc Surg 1:183–6
19. Roe CF (1971) Effect of bowel exposure on body temperature during surgical operations. Am J Surg 122:13–15
20. Seitzinger NM, Dudgeon LS (1993) Decreasing the degree of hypothermia during prolonged laparoscopic procedures. J Reprod Med 38:511–513
21. Sessier DI, Hynson J, McGuire J, Moayeri A, J-Ieier T (1992) Thermoregulatory vasoconstriction during isofluorane anaesthesia minimally decreases heat loss. Anesthesiology 76:670–675
22. Sessler DI (1993) Perianesthetic thermoregulation and heat balance in humans. FASEB J 7:638–644
23. Shanks CA, Ronai AK, Schafer MF (1988) The effects of airway heat conservation and skin surface insulation on thermal balance during spinal surgery. Anesthesiology 69:956–958
24. Sheffield CW, Sessler DI, Hunt TK (1994) Mild hypothermia during isofluorane anesthesia decreases resistance to *E. coli* dermal infection in guinea pigs. Anesth Analg 38(3):201–205
25. Slotman GJ, Jed EH, Burchard KW (1985) Adverse effects of hypothermia in postoperative patients. Am J Surg 149:495–501
26. Stevens WC, Cromwell TH, Halsey MJ, Eger EI, Shakespeare TF, Bahlman SH (1971)The cardiovascular effects of a new inhalational anesthetic, Forane, in human volunteers at constant arterial carbon dioxide tension. Anesthesiology 35:8–16
27. Tollofsrud S, Gunderson Y, Anderson R (1984) Perioperative hypothermia. Acta Anaesthesiol Scand 28:511–515
28. Wallasvaara MP (1992) Ventilation and body temperatures during laparoscopic vs open cholecystectomy. Anesth Analg 74:S340

4 Pneumoperitoneum-Related Circulatory Changes of the Lower Extremities

M.A. REYMOND, Y. CHRISTEN, P. MOREL, and F. KÖCKERLING

Introduction

The peritoneal cavity is a virtual space in which there is a hydrostatic pressure known as the intra-abdominal pressure [1]. Under physiological conditions, e.g. physical effort or defecation, intra-abdominal pressure varies considerably. If this pressure increases for pathophysiological or iatrogenic reasons, hemodynamic changes result. These changes may be acute, e.g., hemorrhage, pneumoperitoneum (PNP), or occur gradually, e.g., ascites. In anatomical terms, the causes may be intraperitoneal or retroperitoneal. Two situations are of particular interest to the surgeon, namely the abdominal compartment syndrome and PNP.

The abdominal compartment syndrome has long been known to pediatric surgeons who have encountered it following surgical correction of omphalocele or gastroschisis. This syndrome was accurately defined by Fietsam [2] on the basis of the following criteria: elevated intra-abdominal pressure, tachycardia, elevated central venous pressure, hypoxia, and hypercapnia. Such syndromes may occur after trauma, for example following severe injury to the vertebral column, or injury to the kidneys. In general surgery, an abdominal compartment syndrome may be caused by the rupture of an aortic aneurysm into the retroperitoneum. Such a syndrome may also develop after the operative repair of large cicatricial hernias or in association with bleeding following retroperitoneal procedures. The danger of an abdominal compartment syndrome has been shown to be directly related to the intra-abdominal pressure, as has been demonstrated in patients in whom continuous measurements were obtained via a catheter in the bladder [3]. If the intra-abdominal pressure exceeds 25 mmHg, surgical decompression must be performed. Pressures of less than 20 mmHg appear not to pose any threat to the patient's life. Until recently little attention has been given to the effects of increased intra-abdominal pressure on the hemodynamics in the lower extremities. However, it may be expected that these effects are, in principle, similar to those produced by PNP, yet are more pronounced.

In this chapter, the effects of PNP on the hemodynamics in the lower extremities are described in detail. This topic is of relevance since venous stasis may predispose to postoperative thromboembolism. Patients undergoing a laparoscopic procedure are anesthetized and are often operated in the reverse-Trendelenburg position with a PNP of 12–15 mmHg. All of these factors can lead to venous stasis, which may favor the occurrence of postoperative deep vein thrombosis. A number of reports of deep vein thromboses [4–9], nonfatal pulmonary embolism [4, 10–12], or even fatal pulmonary embolisms [4] have been published in recent years. How such complications occur and how they can be avoided is best explained by pathophysiological considerations of the influence of PNP on the hemodynamics of the lower extremities.

Experimental Data

In the angiological laboratory, increased extra-abdominal pressure was applied to healthy subjects, and changes in venous hemodynamics of the lower extremities were observed with duplex ultrasound. In addition, the influence of PNP on the venous capacitance and outflow were documented during different surgical procedures by means of plethysmography. In a subsequent step, invasive measurements of pressure were carried out during laparoscopic cholecystectomy. In these studies, the influence of patient positioning and different PNP pressures were investigated [13]. In addition, the question of whether the use of compression stockings could correct the observed disturbances was also investigated [14].

In the first study, the question was investigated as to whether, during laparoscopic cholecystectomy, the venous capacitance and maximum venous outflow are influenced by PNP during laparoscopic cholecystectomy. To this end, seven men and five women with a mean age of 59.7 years were recruited to the study. The measurements were carried out using a pressure plethysmograph prior to, during, and after establishment of a PNP (14 mmHg). Venous stasis was induced using a cuff pressure of 60 mmHg. After calibrating the equipment, the venous capacitance and maximum venous outflow were measured on the basis of standardized criteria. The maximum increase in volume under standard conditions in the presence of venous stasis was defined as the venous capacitance and expressed in arbitrary units. Venous stasis was released abruptly after a volume plateau had been achieved. In this way, the maximum venous outflow in 1 s was calculated. The three measurements (prior to, during, and after PNP) were compared with one another. The statistical analysis was perfomed using two-way analysis of variance (ANOVA; measuring time points and side). In this way, it was demonstrated that a PNP of 14 mmHg restricted the venous capacitance by 19% in the right leg and by 31% in the left leg ($p = 0.006$). However, there were no significant differences to be found between the two extremities. After releasing the PNP, the baseline situation was largely restored (Fig. 1). In a similar manner, PNP also exercises an influence on maximal venous outflow, a decrease of 9% on the right and of 26% on the left being measured. Because of the small number of patients involved in this study, this difference did not reach statistical significance, nor was there any significant difference between the two sides. As in the case of venous capacitance, the baseline figures were again restored after release of the PNP. On the basis of these pneumoplethysmographic measurements, it may be concluded that a PNP of 14 mmHg results in venous stasis in the lower extremities, which is reflected by a reduction in venous capacitance and maximum venous outflow. These changes are more marked in the left limb, as compared with the right, presumably due to anatomical reasons.

In the angiological laboratory, an attempt was made to reproduce conditions similar to those obtained with PNP in the operating theater. A total of 12 male

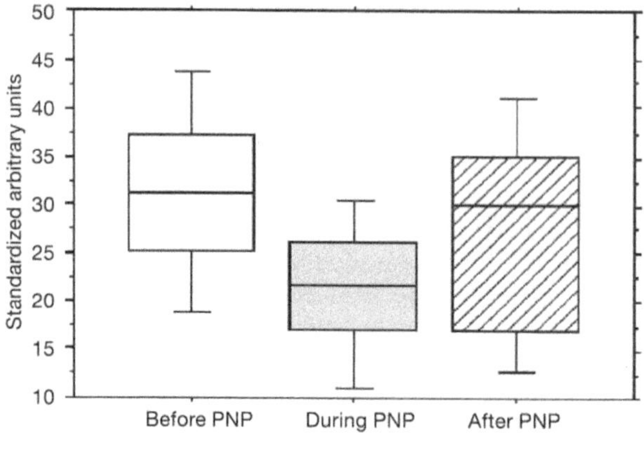

Fig. 1. Venous capacitance before, during, and after application of 14 mmHg pneumoperitoneum (*PNP*) ($p > 0.10$)

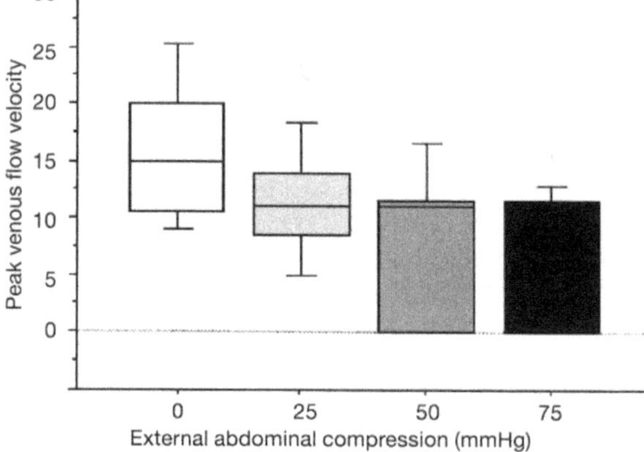

Fig. 2. Venous flow in the common femoral vein during application of progressive extra-abdominal compression ($p < 0.0001$)

subjects with an average age of 34±7 years and an average weight of 70.5 ± 7 kg were investigated. A long, 15-cm-wide cuff applied around the abdomen was inflated under manometric control (Plethysmograph SP2, Medimatic, Denmark). At each pressure step, peak venous flow velocity in the right common femoral vein was investigated using duplex ultrasound (Diasonics DRF-300, 10-MHz probe). Measurements were obtained at pressures of 0, 25, 50, and 75 mmHg. Each patient served as his/her own control. The statistical analysis was carried out as a one-way ANOVA.

A pressure increase from 0 to 75 mmHg resulted in a pronounced decrease in peak venous flow velocity from 16.0 cm/s (range, 9.0–28.0 cm/s) to 7.1 cm/s (range, 0.0–13.0 cm/s) (56%, $p < 0.0001$, Fig. 2). By applying extra-abdominal pressure in healthy subjects we were able to elicit changes in the venous hemodynamics of the lower extremities in the sense of venous stasis. We subsequently employed this model to study the hemodynamic effects of prophylactic measures (see below).

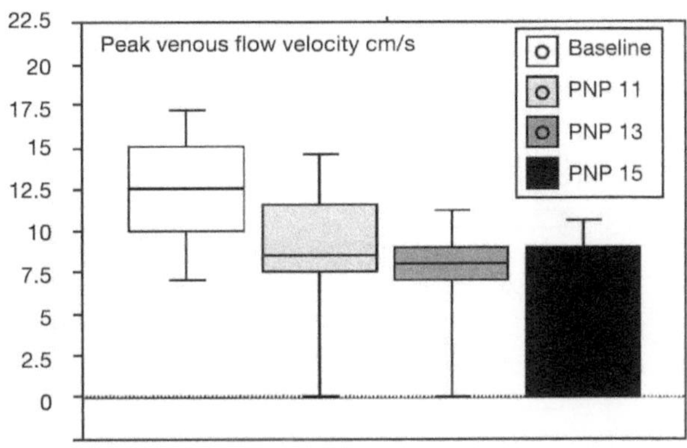

Fig. 3. Effect of increasing pneumoperitoneum (*PNP*) on peak venous flow velocity ($p < 0.0001$)

Changes similar to those found in the above-mentioned study were also established in the operating theater during the establishment of PNP. The hemodynamics in the lower extremities were investigated in seven women and five men (age 53 ± 20 years) undergoing 12 elective laparoscopic cholecystectomies. All of the patients were ASA (American Society of Anesthesiologists) class I or class II and none had a history of thromboembolism. The patients were positioned with their legs spread apart. The measurement of venous flow velocity in the right common femoral vein was monitored by an experienced angiologist using a sterile 7.5-MHz probe connected to an Aloca SSD 650 Duplex-Doppler device. Peak venous flow velocity was calculated automatically by the device. The statistical analysis was performed using two-way ANOVA (PNP and patient position, repeated measures). The peak venous flow velocity decreased from 12.2 ± 4.9 (PNP = 0) to $5.6 + 4.4$ cm/s (PNP = 15) ($p < 0.0001$, Fig. 3). In 50% of the patients, a peak venous flow velocity of less than 6.83 cm/s and a PNP of 15 mmHg were measured. A reduction in PNP pressure from 15 to 11 mmHg resulted in a 54% improvement in peak venous flow velocity ($p = 0.003$). An interesting observation was that the intra-abdominal pressure necessary to reproduce comparable hemodynamic changes in nonanesthetized healthy subjects was considerably lower. The probable explanation for this is that the relaxed abdominal wall of the anesthetized surgical patient no longer plays a role and that the intra-abdominal hydrostatic pressure of the PNP acts directly on the vessel walls. Other authors have reported similar results [15–17], and experiments in the large animal model (swine) also produced identical results, though higher PNP pressures of between 10 and 20 mmHg were required [18].

Under the same conditions as applied to the peak venous flow velocity measurements (see above), the changes in the diameter of the common femoral vein with increasing extra-abdominal pressure were investigated in healthy subjects in the angiological laboratory. The diameter of the femoral vein increased from 12.2 mm (range, 9.2–15.5 mm) initially (baseline) to 14.7 mm (range, 5.5–16.5 mm) at a pressure of 75 mmHg ($p < 0.0001$). In the operating theater the diameter of the common femoral vein increased during laparoscopic cholecystectomies with increasing PNP (Fig. 4). The following values were measured: 9.6 ± 1.6 mm with-

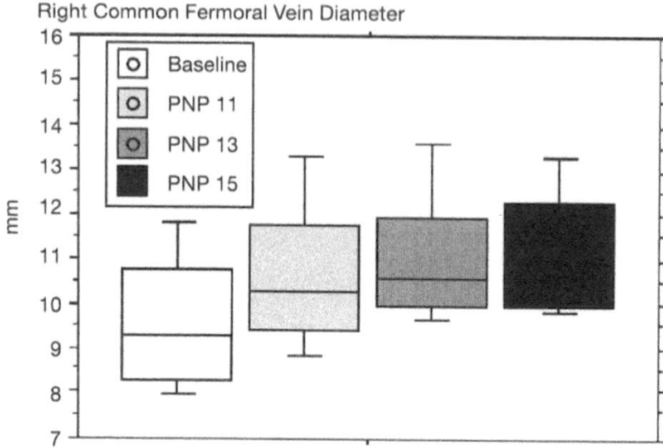

Fig. 4. Effect of increasing pneumoperitoneum (*PNP*) on the diameter of the right common femoral vein ($p < 0.001$)

out PNP and 11.3 ± 1.4 mmwith a PNP of 15 mmHg. Of interest was the observation that an increase in pressure from 13 to 15 mmHg resulted in an increase in the surface area of the vein of only 2% (index 137% to index 139%). These figures show that the femoral vein had already reached peak dilatation at a PNP of 13 mmHg. Ido reported an increase of 184% ± 16.3% in the vessel area at a PNP of 10 mmHg [17]. Beebe noted that a PNP of 14 mmHg banished the pulsatility of the common femoral vein in 75% of the patients, suggesting proximal partial venous obstruction [15]. In all cases the release of PNP was followed by restoration of normal pulsatility. It has been suggested that excessive vasodilatation might give rise to microtears in the vascular endothelium [19]. Whether the PNP-related maximum dilatation of the vessel leads to microscopic lesions in the endothelium is still not clear.

In the same 12 laparoscopic cholecystectomies, we undertook invasive measurements of the pressure in the left common femoral vein. Studies were approved by the relevant ethics committee of the university hospital in Geneva, Switzerland. All patients involved were fully informed and gave their written consent to participate. Pressures were recorded via a 3-F teflon catheter. This catheter was introduced using the Seldinger technique and attached to a Hewlett-Packard quartz transducer (1290C). Anesthesia was standardized and implemented in accordance with an exact protocol – in particular, adequate relaxation was ensured by constant monitoring. Each patient served as his/her own control. Repeated measurements were compared with the baseline figures. In this way it was documented that the pressure in the femoral vein increased parallel to the PNP – from 8.8 ± 4.1 mmHg (baseline) to 18.7 ± 5.5 mmHg (at a PNP pressure of 15 mmHg; Figure 5, $p < 0.001$). When the pressure was reduced from 15 to 11 mmHg, the venous pressure decreased by 20.1% ($p < 0.001$). Similar invasive pressure measurements have been carried out in another study [16]: at a PNP of 14–16 mmHg, the femoral vein pressure was recorded (18.2 ± 5.1 mmHg), again doubling the baseline values.

In contrast to gynecological procedures, laparoscopy in general surgery often requires the patient to be placed in a reverse-Trendelenburg position. This applies in particular to operations involving the upper abdomen (e.g., cholecys-

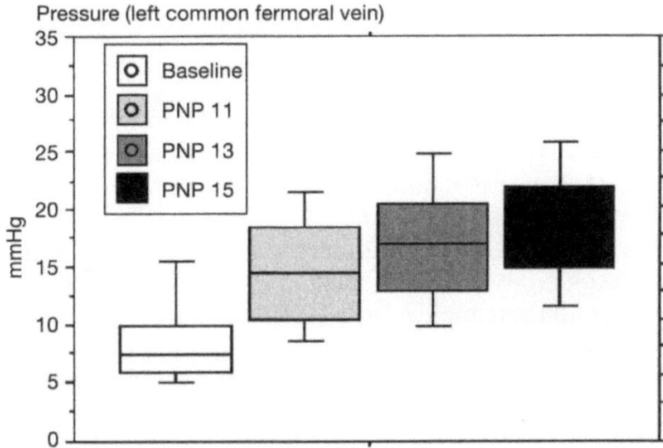

Fig. 5. Effect of increasing pneumoperitoneum (*PNP*) on the pressure in the left common femoral vein ($p < 0.0001$)

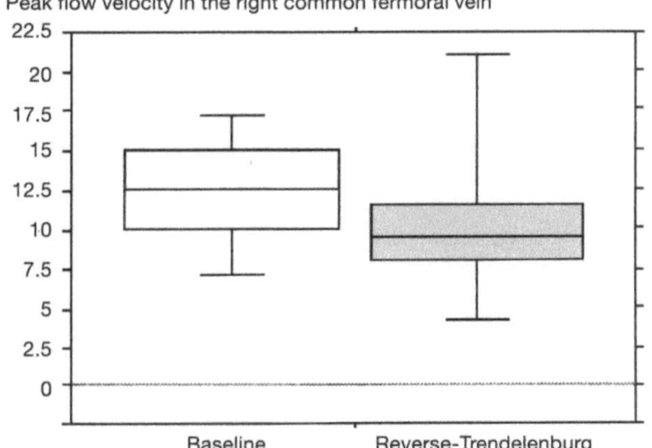

Fig. 6. Effect of reverse-Trendelenburg position on the peak flow velocity in the right common femoral vein ($p = 0.07$)

tectomy and Nissen fundoplication). Under such conditions, it is to be expected that venous stasis in the lower extremities will be increased. During laparoscopic cholecystectomies in the reverse-Trendelenburg position we observed a decrease in the average peak venous flow velocity in the right femoral vein from 12.3 ± 4.9 to 10.5 ± 5.8 cm/s (Fig. 6). Since considerable differences were observed between patients, these values did not reach statistical significance ($p = 0.07$). The mean pressure also decreased from 8.8 mmHg to 3.5 mmHg ($p < 0.001$). This negative difference can be explained by the fact that the point of measurement is located in the groin, and in the reverse-Trendelenburg position is higher than the patient's feet. Also, the diameter of the femoral vein changed significantly in this position, from 9.6 ± 1.6 mm to 10.3 ± 1.8 mm ($p = 0.004$). Similar results were reported in two other studies [17, 18].

Our knowledge about postoperative disturbances in the composition of the blood has greatly improved in recent years. A disturbance in the homeostasis of the coagulation system resulting in hypercoagulability increases the likelihood of a thromboembolic event to occur [20]. Caprini investigated whole blood by thrombelastography (TEG) and plasma activated partial thromboplastin time (PTT) on the first postoperative day in 100 patients undergoing laparoscopic cholecystectomy. All the patients received preoperative, intraoperative and postoperative mechanical prophylaxis. Of these, 36 patients with an elevated thrombosis risk received additional prophylaxis with heparin over a period of 4 weeks. They concluded that both the TEG index ($p = 0.005$) and the PTT ($p = 0.05$) had undergone a change indicative of hypercoagulability [10]. In another study, fibrinogen, cross-linked fibrin degradation products (D-dimer), prothrombin international normalized ratio (INR), activated PTT, and platelets were measured prior to, during, and after open (seven patients) and laparoscopic (13 patients) Nissen fundoplication procedures. In both groups, the postoperative fibrinogen levels increased significantly, while the other coagulation parameters remained unchanged [21].

Both Jorgensen in animal experimental studies [18] and Goodale in patients [16] were unable to find any adaptation of the hemodynamics of the lower extremities during lengthy laparoscopic procedures involving PNP. We ourselves did not investigate the question of adaptability.

Clinical Data

The above-mentioned experimental observations in patients and in animal experiments have clear theoretical consequences with respect to the potential development of postoperative deep venous thrombosis and pulmonary embolism. In 1856, Virchow recognized three possible causes underlying a thrombosis: changes in vessel walls, in the blood flow, and in the composition of the blood [22]. Postoperative thromboembolism is a feared complication of conventional abdominal surgery, too. Long operating times, carcinomas, and other factors all favor development of a thrombosis. In conventional surgery, the clinical signs of deep vein thrombosis or a pulmonary embolism usually occur in the second postoperative week [20]. As a rule, postoperative deep vein thromboses are distant thrombotic events which, irrespective of the surgical field, occur in the patient's lower extremities. The point of origin of these deep vein thromboses is found most often in the deep veins of the calf. In contrast, a pulmonary embolism is usually a result of an upper leg or pelvic vein thrombosis. For intra-abdominal procedures, the risk of deep vein thrombosis occurring is reported to be about 25% in patients older than 40 years when no specific antithrombotic prophylaxis has been employed [23, 24]. Following conventional cholecystectomy under prophylactic cover, the incidence of deep vein thrombosis as assessed by phlebography has been found to be 10% [19]. In this group of surgical patients, a risk of pulmonary embolism of 0.4%–7% has been reported [25, 26].

To date, few clinical data have been published on the incidence of such events after laparoscopic surgery, and most benign deep vein thromboses will go unnoticed clinically if no specific diagnostic search is undertaken (e.g., phlebography, duplex sonography, D-dimers, plethysmography). Since laparoscopic surgery is associated with only a short stay in the hospital, there is a potential danger that these complications may occur only after patient discharge and will therefore not be recorded. Data presently available stem either from large data banks, where the information is often imprecise, or from small groups of patients where, although the information is accurate, conclusions may not be drawn on account of the small numbers involved. It is also difficult to determine what medical and/or physical prophylactic measures were employed, and when preoperative, intraoperative, postoperative, or combinations were applied. The incidence of deep vein thrombosis and pulmonary embolism after diagnostic gynecological laparoscopy appears to be low. Thus, in a study involving 50,427 patients, an incidence of thromboembolic events of 0.02% cases undergoing such procedures was reported [27]. Among a total of 438 laparoscopic cholecystectomies, three deep vein thromboses, one fatal and one nonfatal pulmonary embolism were observed. This represents an incidence of 0.64% in the case of deep vein thrombosis, and 0.45% in the case of pulmonary embolism [4]. Among 230 laparoscopic fundoplications, Watson observed four cases of pulmonary embolism [12]. Mayol reported two cases of nonfatal pulmonary embolism following 200 cholecystectomies, but did not provide any information about the incidence of deep vein thrombosis [11]. Ido observed a single pulmonary embolism among 850 laparoscopic cholecystectomies [17]. In a multicenter prospective study "Laparoscopic Colorectal Surgery" undertaken in German-speaking European countries, no case of deep vein thrombosis or pulmonary embolism was observed after 504 procedures [28]. The study done by Caprini is the only one in which a postoperative examination was routinely carried out [10]. Among 103 cases of cholecystectomy examined by duplex ultrasonography of the lower limbs 1 week after surgery, a single case of deep vein thrombosis was noted. None of these patients were observed to have clinical pulmonary embolism.

The above-mentioned data from our own studies and those obtained from the literature show that at least two of the three factors in Virchow's triad – venous stasis and hypercoagulability – are present during and following laparoscopic procedures. For this reason, the surgeon must consider using thromboprophylaxis. The prophylactic measures applied worldwide for the prevention of thromboembolic events are the use of heparin and mechanical measures: heparin to prevent hypercoagulability and mechanical measures to prevent intraoperative and postoperative stasis.

The introduction of low molecular weight heparins in the middle of the 1980s represented a major development of conventional heparin prophylaxis in which, as a result of molecular fractionation, the anticoagulatory factor (factor X) was improved vis-à-vis the antithrombotic factor (factor II A).

As a result of the doubling of the biological half-life of the fractionated heparin molecule, the use of the low molecular weight heparins made it possible to achieve antithrombotic prophylaxis with a single daily injection, thus making it highly practical in both the hospital and outpatient settings. With respect to the undesired side effect of bleeding, carefully implemented controlled studies on low molecular weight heparins have revealed no increase despite the improvement in their effectiveness profile. However, at this point, it should be noted that on release of the PNP, venous bleeding may increase, since the pressure gradient between the intravascular compartment and the abdominal cavity increases abruptly.

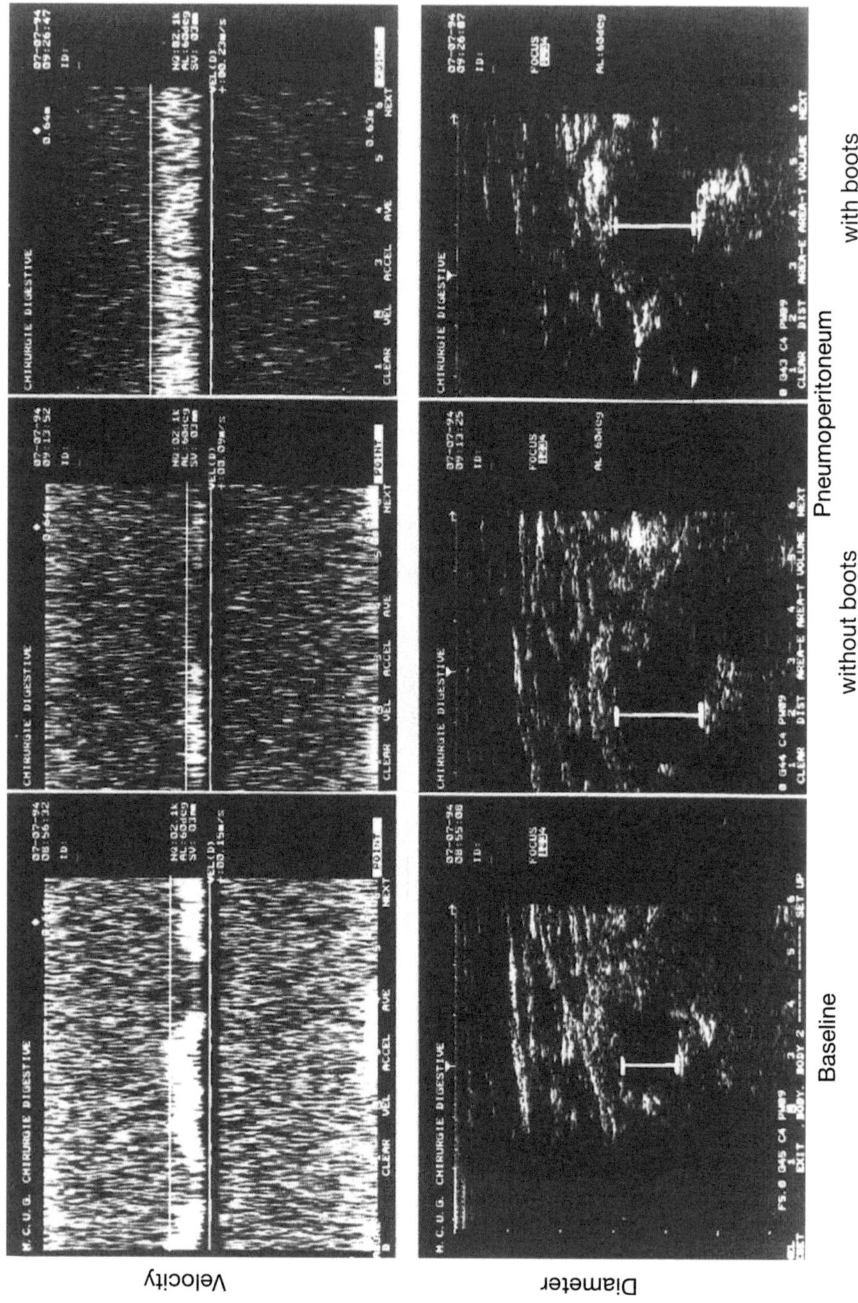

Fig. 7. Effect of compression devices on venous flow velocity (*upper pictures*) and on the diameter of the common femoral vein (*lower pictures*)

In our own patient population and in healthy subjects, we have investigated the hemodynamic effects of sequential compression of the lower limbs using compression boots. For this purpose, the diameter and peak blood flow in the right common femoral vein were measured in the angiological laboratory and during laparoscopic cholecystectomy. The invasive pressure could, of course, be measured only during the surgical procedure (see above). The results of the measurements with and without the use of compression boots were compared. Each patient acted as his/her own control. The null hypothesis was that the boots would have no effect. The differences found were tested with one-way ANOVA. In both patients and healthy subjects, intermittent compression using the boots restored the peak venous flow velocity, which had been greatly reduced by hydrostatic pressure (Fig. 7). However, neither the original diameter of the vein nor the original pressure was restored [14]. It was thus established that, although intermittent compression restored femoral venous flow, the venous high-pressure state caused by the PNP could be overcome only by higher pressures.

Similar findings were reported by Jorgensen [8], who investigated the effect of two mechanical methods of prophylaxis. Intermittent pneumatic compression (IPC) and intermittent electrical calf stimulation (IECS) were used with a PNP of 12 mmHg. Both methods restored pulsatile flow, but proved to have no influence on the reduced baseline venous flow velocity – a certain degree of stasis thus persisted. Wilson investigated the use of static compression stockings in cholecystectomy procedures [29]. The venous capacitance and maximal venous outflow were measured with the aid of plethysmography. In the group not wearing compression stockings, both parameters were reduced in the majority of patients. In the group wearing static stockings, the venous PNP-induced changes were less marked or not even measurable. The intraoperative measurements revealed a significant difference favoring the group wearing the stockings. A fourth mechanical method of prophylaxis makes use of compression leg bandages [17]. This method was able to restore venous flow only with PNP pressures below 5 mmHg.

Conclusions

It cannot be denied that thromboembolic events can occur after laparoscopic procedures. The fact that such complications occur relatively early in the post-operative phase suggests an intraoperative etiology. Experimental findings are also compatible with acute intraoperative venous stasis. In contrast to gynecological procedures, most general surgical laparoscopic interventions are performed with the patient in a reverse-Trendelenburg position, which additionally favors venous stasis. Further risk factors include prolonged operating times and tumor surgery such as, for example, colorectal procedures or pelvic lymphadenectomy in gynecological or prostate cancers. Obese patients are at increased risk. On the basis of the data collected to date, the incidence of deep vein thromboses and pulmonary embolism would appear to be lower than that observed in comparable conventional procedures, although reliable randomized data are still not yet available. This lower incidence might be explained by less surgical tissue damage and earlier postoperative mobilization. Various reports of complications do, however, show that in the absence of prophylactic antithrombotic measures, laparoscopic interventions are not without risk. For these reasons, the recommendations of a Consensus Conference [23] and relevant guidelines [34] require the application of antithrombotic measures in laparoscopic surgery, too. The PNP pressure can often be maintained at a low level. After operations in the reverse-Trendelenburg position, the patient should be brought back into a neutral position as quickly as possible. Although mechanical prophylactic measures are to be recommended, they do not suffice to ensure the patient's safety when used alone. Until randomized prospective studies show otherwise, aggressive antithrombosis measures must be instituted in all patients undergoing laparscopic surgery as they are in conventional surgery

Summary

How great is the actual risk of postoperative thromboembolic events following laparoscopic procedures (Fig. 8)? Although the above-mentioned studies permit only tentative conclusions to be drawn as to the incidence of thromboembolic complications, it would not appear to be particularly high, and is probably lower than that associated with conventional surgery. The question as to how this lower incidence is compatible with the experimental venous stasis and hypercoagulability remains unanswered. Other factors, for example, faster mobilization of the patient, must presumably also play an important role. It is interesting

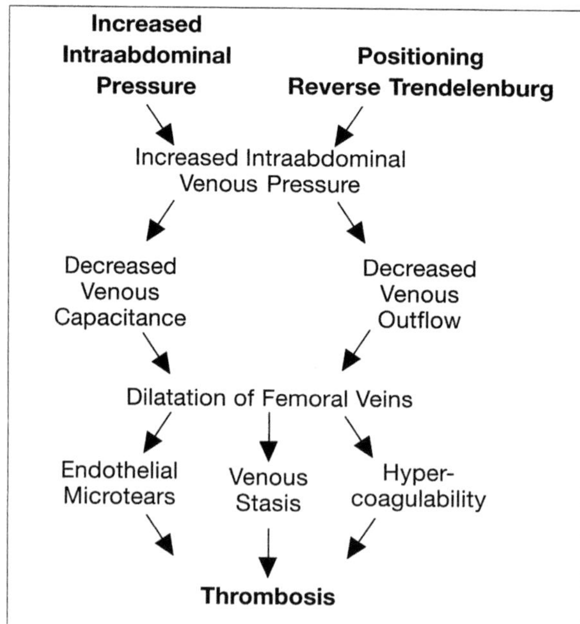

Fig. 8. Algorithm of pneumoperitoneum and thrombosis

to note that possible thromboembolic events appear to occur earlier after laparoscopic (third to fifth postoperative day) than after conventional surgery (typically in the second postoperative week), which would suggest an intraoperative etiology. Prospective studies involving routine postoperative examinations would certainly be helpful. A study involving routine postoperative phlebography in asymptomatic patients would be problematic, since this radiological method is associated with pain, radiation exposure, and potential risks. Although the sensitivity of echo Doppler ultrasound is lower, such an examination would be far more acceptable to the patient.

It is important to emphasize that a number of different factors are associated with an elevated risk of thromboembolism (Table 1). These risk factors are patient illness- and operation-related. Obese patients are those most likely to benefit from the laparoscopic approach [30–32], there being fewer postoperative complications, in particular fewer thromboembolic events, in comparison with open surgery [17]. It is nevertheless a known fact that overweight patients undergoing open surgery more often develop postoperative thrombosis. Older age and smoking are additional risk factors. In the case of women, pregnancy and the use of oral contraceptives favor the development of thrombi. A history of thromboembolic events increases the risk by a factor of two to three. Malignant diseases, cardiovascular diseases, in particular right-sided heart failure, and varicosis, are all illness-related factors. In addition, hypercoagulability (antithrombin III, protein C or protein S deficiency, the antiphospholipid syndrome, reduced plasminogen activator inhibitor, polycythemia vera) all increase the risk of thrombosis. It was earlier feared that prolonged laparoscopic procedures (lasting more than 90 min) would be associated with an elevated risk of thrombosis. In the case of colorectal procedures, however, this expected high incidence of such events did not materialize, possibly because appropriate prophylactic measures were taken and patients were operated on in the Trendelenburg position. A prolonged reverse-Trendelenburg position and a high PNP pressure are also potentially dangerous. It must be supposed that splenectomy and procedures in the pelvis are, as in the case of open surgery, associated with an elevated risk of thrombosis.

For conventional surgery, it has been shown that mechanical prophylactic measures not only have a positive hemodynamic effect, but that they also actually do reduce the incidence of deep venous thrombosis [33]. The use of mechanical prophylactic measures in laparoscopic procedures is logical, since experimental

Table 1. Risk factors for thromboembolic events following laparoscopic surgery

Patient	Disease	Procedure
Age over 45	Carcinoma	Duration (> 90 min)
History of thromboembolism	Hypercoagulability	Prolonged reverse –
	Varicosis	Trendelenburg position
Obesity	Cardiovascular	High pneumoperitoneum
	disorders	pressure (> 13 mmHG)
Pregnancy		Splenectomy
Use of oral contraceptives		Surgery in the pelvis
Smoking		(e.g., lymphadenectomy)

work has adequately shown that such mechanical measures can at least partially correct the undesired hemodynamic side effects of PNP. IPC and IECS must therefore be considered effective mechanical prophylaxis. Compression stockings, in contrast, are only of limited application, since they are employed in a static high-pressure system. However, they may be of advantage in the postoperative phase. Compression leg bandages, however, are ineffective under clinical conditions and should not be used.

Even when additional mechanical prophylactic measures have been applied, medical prophylaxis must also be given, since surgical hypercoagulability persists for at least 8–10 days. This makes prophylactic medication, where applicable on an outpatient basis, necessary [34]. As in the case of any other medication, a cost–benefit analysis of such antithrombotic prophylaxis should be carried out. To date, however, such an analysis has not been undertaken for laparoscopic surgery.

References

1. Overholt RH (1931) Intraperitoneal pressure. Arch Surg 22:691–703
2. Fietsam R, Villalba M, Glover JR, Clark K (1989) Intraabdominal compartment syndrome as a complication of ruptured intraabdominal aneurysm repair. Am Surg 55:396–402
3. Kron IL, Harman K, Nolan SP (1984) The measurement of intraabdominal pressure as a criterion for abdominal reexploration. Ann Surg 199:28–30
4. Jorgensen JO, Hanel K, Lalak NJ, Hunt DR, North L, Morris DL (1993) Thromboembolic complications of laparoscopic cholecystectomy. BMJ 306:518–519
5. Deziel DJ, Millikan KW, Economou SG, Doolas A, Ko ST, Airan MC (1993) Complications of laparoscopic cholecystectomy: a national survey of 4292 hospitals and an analysis of 77 604 cases. Am J Surg 165:9–14
6. Airan M, Appel M, Berci G, Coburg AJ, Cohen M, Cuschieri A, Dent T, Duppler D, Easter D, Greene F et al (1992) Retrospective and prospective multi-institutional laparoscopic cholecystectomy study organized by the Society of American Gastrointestinal Endoscopic Surgeons. Surg Endosc 6:169–176
7. Dubois F, Berthelot G, Levard H (1991) Laparoscopic cholecystectomy: historic perspective and personal experience. Surg Laparosc Endosc 1:52–57
8. Jorgensen JO, Lalak NJ, North L, Hanel K, Hunt DR, Morris DL (1994) Venous stasis during laparoscopic cholecystectomy. Surg Laparosc Endosc 4:128–133
9. Scott TR, Zucker KA, Bailey RW (1992) Laparoscopic cholecystectomy: a review of 12 397 patients. Surg Laparosc Endosc 2:191–198
10. Caprini JA, Areelus JI, Laubach M, Size G, Hoffman KN, Coats RW, Blattner S (1995) Postoperative hypercoagulability and deep-vein thrombosis after laparoscopic cholecystectomy. Surg Endosc 9:304–309
11. Mayol J, Vincent-Hamelin E, Sarmiento JM, Oshiro EO, Diaz-Gonzalez J, Tamayo FJ, Fernandez-Represa JA (1994) Pulmonary embolism following laparoscopic cholecystectomy: report of two cases and review of the literature. Surg Endosc 8:214–217
12. Watson DI, Jamieson GG, Devitt PG, Matthew G, Britten-Jones RE, Game PA, Williams RS (1995) Changing strategies in the performance of laparoscopic Nissen fundoplication as a result of experience with 230 operations. Surg Endosc 9:961–966
13. Reymond MA, Christen Y, Klopfenstein C, Tassile D, Bounameaux H, Morel P (1995) Influence of pneumoperitoneum and reverse Trendelenburg position on the venous return during laparoscopic cholecystectomy. HBP Surg 9(S5):15
14. Christen Y, Reymond MA, Vogel JJ, Klopfenstein CE, Morel P, Bounameaux H (1995) Hemodynamic effects of intermittent pneumatic compression of the lower limbs during laparoscopic cholecystectomy. Am J Surg 170:395–398

15. Beebe DS, McNevin MP, Crain JM, Letourneau JG, Belani KG, Abrams JA, Goodale RL (1993) Evidence of venous stasis after abdominal insufflation for laparoscopic cholecystectomy. Surg Gynecol Obstet 176:443–447

16. Goodale RL, Beebe DS, McNevin MP, Boyle M, Letourneau JG, Abrams JH, Cerra FB (1993) Hemodynamic, respiratory, and metabolic effects of laparoscopic cholecystectomy. Am J Surg 166:533–537

17. Ido K, Suzuki T, Taniguchi Y, Kawamoto C, Isoda N, Nagamine N, Loka T, Kimura M, Kumagai M, Hirayama Y (1995) Femoral vein stasis during laparoscopic cholecystectomy: effects of graded elastic compression leg bandages in preventing thrombus formation. Gastrointest Endosc 42:151–155

18. Jorgensen JO, Gillies RB, Lalak NJ, Hunt DR (1994) Lower limb venous hemodynamics during laparoscopy: an animal study. Surg Laparosc Endosc 4:32–35

19. Comerota AJ, Stewart GJ, White JV (1985) Combined dihydroergotamine and heparin prophylaxis of postoperative deep vein thrombosis: proposed mechanism of action. Am J Surg 150:39–44

20. Ratschow M, Heberer G, Rau G, Schoop W (1974) Angiologie. Grundlagen, Klinik und Praxis. Thieme, Stuttgart, pp 7217–7225

21. Pike GI, Bessell JR, Mathew G, Watson DI, Mitchell PC, Jamieson E (1996) Changes in fibrinogen levels in patients undergoing open and laparoscopic Nissen fundoplication. Aust N Z J Surg 66:94–96

22. Virchow R (1856) Gesammelte Abhandlungen zur Wissenschaftlichen Medicin. Berlin

23. National Institute of Health (1986) Consensus conference on prevention of venous thrombosis and pulmonary embolism. JAMA 256:744–748

24. Colditz GA, Turden RL, Oster G (1986) Rates of venous thrombosis after general surgery: combined results of randomized clinical trials. Lancet 2:143–146

25. Haas S, Flosbach CW (1990) Prevention of postoperative thromboembolism in general surgery with enoxaparin: preliminary findings. Acta Chir Scand 156:96–102

26. Huber A, Bounameaux H, Borst F, Rohner A (1992) Postoperative pulmonary embolism after hospital discharge: an underestimated risk. Arch Surg 127:310–313

27. Chamberlain G, Brown JC (1978) Gynecological laparoscopy. The report of a working party in a confidential inquiry of gynecological laparoscopy. Royal College of Obstetricians and Gynaecologists, London

28. Kockerling F, Schneider C, Reymond MA, Scheidbach H, Wittekind C, Colorectal Laparoscopic Surgery Study Group (1996) Laparoscopic colorectal surgery: a prospective multicenter trial. Surg Endosc 10:559

29. Wilson YG, Allen PE, Skidmore R, Baker AR (1994) Influence of compression stockings on lower-limb venous hemodynamics during laparoscopic cholecystectomy. Br J Surg 81:841–844

30. Miles RH, Carballo RE, Prinz RA, McMahon M, Pulawski G, Olen RN, Dahlinghaus DL (1992) Laparoscopy: the preferred method of cholecystectomy in the morbidly obese. Surgery 112:818–822

31. Schirmer BD, Dix J, Edge SB, Hyser MJ, Hanks JB, Aguilar M (1992) Laparoscopic cholecystectomy in the obese patient. Ann Surg 216:146–152

32. Collet D, Edye M, Magne E, Perissat J (1992) Laparoscopic cholecystectomy in the obese patient. Surg Endosc 6:186–188

33. Nicolaides AN, Fernandes J, Pollock AV (1980) Intermittent sequential pneumatic compression of the legs in the prevention of venous stasis and postoperative deep venous thrombosis. Surgery 87:69–76

34. Koppenhagen K, Hiiring R (1995) Aktuelle Aspekte zur stationaren und ambulanten Thromboembolie-Prophylaxe. In: Deutsche Gesellschaft fur Chirurgie (ed) Grundlagen der Chirurgie, G66. Demeter, Balingen

5 Influence of Increased Intra-abdominal Pressure on the Hepatoportal Circulation

J. Martz and M. Shimizu

Introduction

Laparoscopy results in an increase in intra-abdominal pressure (IAP). Increased IAP is seen, not only in a multitude of other clinical situations, but also as a result of bowel distention secondary to ileus or mechanical obstruction. It is seen in trauma, with intraperitoneal or retroperitoneal bleeding, in bowel distention from massive resuscitation efforts, in abdominal packing for control of persistent bleeding, and as a result of the application of military anti-shock trousers (MAST) [1]. Increased IAP is also seen in some chronic conditions such as liver failure with resultant ascites [2]. The effects of increased IAP on liver function and hepatic and portal blood flow will be discussed below.

Physiology

The acute effects of increased IAP and its effects on hepatic blood flow have been studied for nearly 100 years. Increasing abdominal pressure results in increased resistance to prograde flow in the abdominal vasculature. Thus an incremental increased pressure is necessary to perfuse visceral organs including the liver, kidney, and mesentery [1]. Researchers have studied the resistance of hepatic blood flow for nearly 70 years. By applying the following formula, they calculated a resistance in the portal vein of 0.0174 mmHg and in the hepatic artery of 1.14 mmHg [3].

$$R = A\text{-}V/F$$, where R is resistance, A-V is the difference in pressure, and F is the blood flow.

The diminished blood flow in the portal vasculature and its concomitant histopathological changes consistent with liver dysfunction, as a result of increased IAP, have been well studied [3].

Bile production has also been considered a measure of hepatic function. Much of the original research on bile production lead to the discovery that increased portal blood flow resulted in increased bile production. Studies have shown that the stimulation of increased portal blood flow in dogs resulted in an increased flow of bile. Similarly, when portal venous flow was excluded, bile secretion ceased [3].

In regard to total blood flow of the liver, the hepatic artery is responsible for 25%–30% of it. However, there is an inverse relationship between blood flow in the portal system and the hepatic artery. Increased hepatic artery blood flow was seen with occlusions of the portal vein [3].

CO$_2$ Pneumoperitoneum and Hepatoportal Circulation

Recently, the effects of laparoscopy and its associated increased IAP have generated several experimental models (Table 1) [4–6].

Table 1. Experimental models of intra-abdominal pressure (IAP) and its effect on hepatic blood flow

Study	Effects of increased IAP			
Kotzampassi [4] (14 mmHG)	↑ PVP	↓ IVCP	↓ JMBF	
Shuto [5] (8–20 mmHG)	↑ PVP	↑ IVCP	↓ LBF	↓ RBF
Ishizaki [6] (16 mmHG)	↑ PVP	↑ IVCP	↓ THF	↓ SMAF
Diebel [7] (10–40 mmHG)	↑ PVP	↓ HABF	↓ PVBF	↓ HMCBF

PVP, portal venous pressure; IVCP, inferior vena cava pressure; JMBF, jejunal mucosal blood flow; LBF, liver blood flow; RBF; renal blood flow; THF, total hepatic flow; SMAF, superior mesenteric artery flow; HABF, hepatic artery blood flow; PVBF, portal venous blood flow; HMCBF, hepatic microcirculatory blood flow.

Diebel et al. studied the effects of increased IAP on hepatic perfusion in pigs. Their results showed significant reductions in hepatic blood flow with increasing IAP [7]. The changes noted for hepatic microcirculatory blood flow (HMCBF) were affected more by changes in portal venous blood flow (PVBF) than by changes in hepatic artery blood flow (HABF). These differences in liver blood flow to changes in portal inflow that occurred secondary to the increased mechanical compression of the mesenteric vasculature. As described by Richardson et al. there are three major determinants of liver blood flow [8]. These are the hepatic arterial vascular resistance, the mesenteric vascular resistance, and the intrahepatic portal vascular resistance. Under circumstances of elevated IAP, mesenteric vascular resistance can become the major determinant of liver blood flow. Poiseuille's law states that the rate of flow through a tube is proportional to the fourth power of its radius [9]. Therefore, the reduction in the diameter of a mesenteric vein by one half would decrease the flow rate to one sixteenth. It was noted that HABF had a more negative correlation coefficient with IAP than PVBF [7] (Table 2). This may be associated with hormonal influences, including catecholamines and angiotensin, on liver blood flow [10]. Elevated levels of

Table 2. Correlation coefficient between changes in intra-abdominal pressure (IAP) and changes in hepatic artery blood flow (HABF), portal vein blood flow (PVBF), hepatic microcirculatory blood flow (HMCBF), portal venous pressure (PVP) and cardiac output (CO)

Change	Correlation coefficient
△HABF	-0.80*
△PVBF	-0.69*
△HMCBF	-0.85*
PVP	0.96*
△CO	-0.2

*p<0.01.

vasopressin were found in women undergoing laparoscopic gynecological procedures. Vasopressin is a known vasoconstrictor of the renal, celiac, and superior mesenteric vasculature [11].

The role of hypercapnia must also be considered when evaluating the effects of laparoscopy on liver blood flow. Epstein et al. showed significant reductions in hepatic blood flow, splanchnic blood volume, and calculated splanchnic vas-

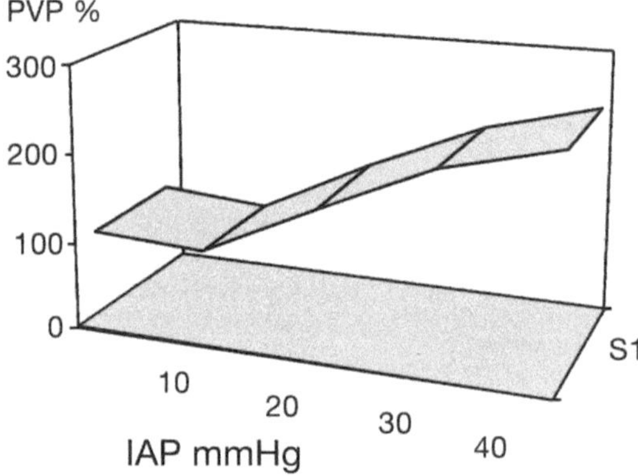

Fig. 1. Intra-abdominal pressure (*IAP*) and portal vein pressure (*PVP*)

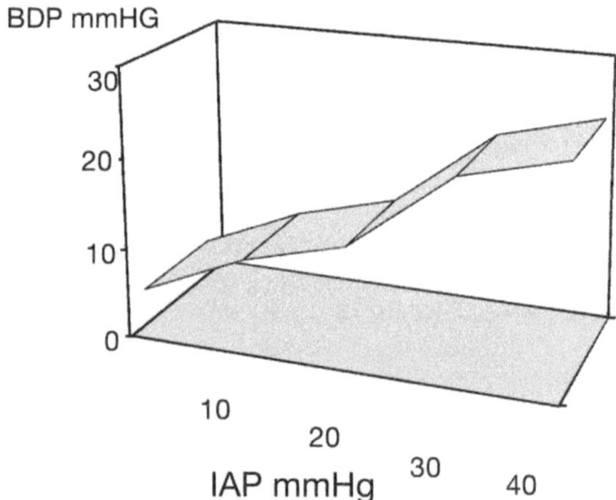

Fig. 2. Intra-abdominal pressure (*IAP*) and bile duct pressure (*BDP*)

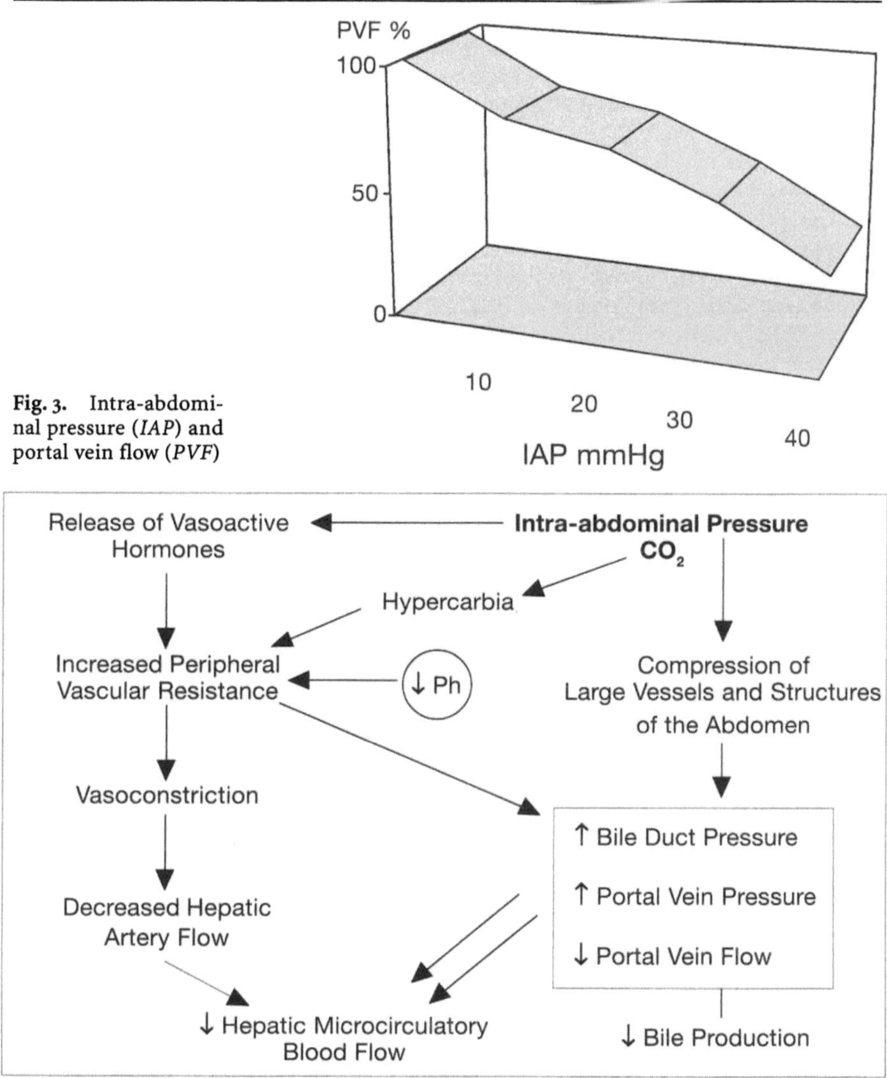

Fig. 3. Intra-abdominal pressure (*IAP*) and portal vein flow (*PVF*)

Fig. 4. Effects of elevated intra-abdominal pressure on the liver caused by direct mechanical pressure

cular resistance. These effects are believed to be mediated by a vasoconstrictive response to elevated carbon dioxide levels in the mesenteric blood [12]. This mechanism, however, appears to be mediated by the central nervous system [13]. Under the influence of elevated PCO_2, denervated splanchnic blood vessels result in splanchnic vasodilatation, not vasoconstriction. This reflex is not affected by neuromuscular blockade.

Shimizu et al. considered in their investigations the effects of elevated IAP on portal venous pressure (PVP), portal venous blood flow (PVBF), and bile duct pressure (BDP) [14]. Elevated IAP was induced in a canine model by the infusion of a starch colloid into the peritoneal cavity. For an IAP of between 0 and 20 mmHg, no statistical difference for PVP and BDP was found. However, for IAP greater than 30 mmHg, a significant elevation ($p < 0.05$) in PVP and BDP was found (Figs. 1, 2,). Similarly, a significantly negative correlation ($p < 0.02$) was discovered between increasing IAP and PVF (Fig. 3). Shimizu concluded that the effects of elevated IAP on the liver are caused by direct mechanical pressure. The compression of the visceral vasculature and bile collecting system will result in decreased flow in their respective systems, and will thus result in liver dysfunction (Fig. 4).

The studies of the effects of elevated IAP by Caldwell reflect the quantitative changes in visceral blood flow [15]. Significant reductions in visceral blood flow were seen at 20 mmHg and 40 mmHg. The adrenal gland, surprisingly, was the exception and retained its blood supply at elevated IAP. The liver showed a significant reduction in blood flow at 20 mmHg ($p < 0.05$) and at 40 mmHg ($p < 0.01$).

Alternative Gases and Hepatoportal Circulation

In another experimental model performed by Sala-Blanch et al. [16], the effect of carbon dioxide and helium pneumoperitoneum on hepatic blood flow was studied. The reduction of hepatic blood flow measured by hepatic extraction of indocyanine green was higher in the helium group than in the CO_2 group (58% vs. 33% reduction). The suprahepatic vein oxygen content ($CshO_2$) value, observed after 90 min of pneumoperitoneum (T1) in the helium group, was lower than the $CshO_2$ levels obtained in the CO_2 group. These authors concluded that a local vasodilator effect of CO_2 could have a theoretical beneficial influence on splanchnic territory in laparoscopic procedures. The elevation of PCO_2 associated with carbon dioxide insufflation may induce sympathetic nervous system changes and thereby lead to vasodilator effects which are intended to "protect" the hepatic blood flow.

Abdominal Compartment Syndrome and Hepatoportal Circulation

The concept of the abdominal compartment syndrome (ACS) as described by Schein et al. [17] can be applied to many clinical circumstances. While laparoscopy may be considered a somewhat transient acute ACS, other clinical scenarios can cause significantly prolonged elevations of IAP. The physiological and clinical effects of changes in volume of the intra-abdominal contents and its resulting changes in IAP have much bearing on laparoscopic surgery [17]. The effects of increased IAP on renal function have been studied in depth [18]. Richards [19] described several clinical examples of acute renal failure in association with elevated IAP. The mechanism he describes is multifactorial, including mechanical compression of the kidneys and their vasculature, and hormonal influences. Similarly increased IAP has been shown to result in liver dysfunction. As described by Lieberman et al. [20], the mass effect of an expanding abdominal aortic aneurysm resulted in compression of the bile outflow.

Elevation in IAP may be considered to result in a mechanically mediated dysfunction of both the liver and many other visceral organs, including the kidneys, spleen, stomach, and intestines. For example, the hepatorenal syndrome may be triggered by the compression of the liver and renal vasculature by an elevated IAP. Consideration of this hypothesis by Savino et al. [21] showed significant improvement in hemodynamics, including cardiac index, stroke index, and significant reductions in blood urea nitrogen (BUN) and creatinine by reducing IAP in cirrhotic patients with acute variceal bleeding.

Conclusions

The effects of elevated intra-abdominal pressure on hepatoportal blood flow have been well studied. The reduction of portal vein and hepatic artery flow is mediated by many influences. Although the effects of direct mechanical compression of the mesenteric vasculature can not be overlooked, other influences must also play a role. These include the affects of hypercarbia, decreased pH, and the role of the many vasoactive hormones. Further opportunities exist for the investigation of these end organ results of elevated IAP.

References

1. Cullen DJ, Coyle JP, Teplick R, Long MC (1989) Cardiovascular, pulmonary, and renal effects of massively increased intra-abdominal pressure in critically ill patients. Crit Care Med 17:118–121
2. Luca A, Cirera I, Garcia-Pagan J, Feu F, Pizcuetta P, Bosch J, Rodes J (1993) Hemodynamic effects of acute changes in intra-abdominal pressure in patients with cirrhosis. Gastroenterology 104:222–227
3. Olerud S (1953) Experimental studies on portal circulation at increased intra-abdominal pressure. Acta Physiol Scand 30 [Suppl 109]:1–95
4. Kotzampassi K, Kapanidis N, Kazamias P, Eleftheriadis E (1993) Hemodynamic events in the peritoneal environment during pneumoperitoneum in dogs. Surg Endosc 7:494–499
5. Shuto K, Kitano S, Yoshida T, Bandoh T, Mitarai Y, Kobayashi M (1995) Hemodynamic and arterial blood gas changes during carbon dioxide and helium pneumoperitoneum in pigs. Surg Endosc 9:1173–1178
6. Ishizaki Y, Bandai Y, Shimonura K, Abe H, Ohtomo Y, Idezuki Y (1993) Changes in splanchnic blood flow and cardiovascular effects following peritoneal insufflation of carbon dioxide. Surg Endosc 7:420–423
7. Diebel LN, Wilson RF, Dulchavsky SA, Saxe J (1992) Effect of increased intra-abdominal pressure on hepatic arterial, portal venous, and hepatic microcirculatory blood flow. J Trauma 33:279–283
8. Richardson PD, Withrington PG (1981) Liver blood flow. Intrinsic and nervous control of liver blood flow. Gastroenterology 81:159–173
9. Damask AC (1978) Medical physics. Physiological physics, external probes. Academic, New York
10. Richardson PD, Withrington PG (1981) Liver blood flow. Effects of drugs and hormones on liver blood flow. Gastroenterology 81:356
11. Punnonen R, Viinamaki O (1982) Vasopressin release during laparoscopy: role of increased intra-abdominal pressure. Lancet 8264:175–176

12. Epstein RM, Wheeler HO, Frumin J, Habif DV, Papper EM, Bradley SE (1961) The effect of hypercapnia on estimated hepatic blood flow, circulating splanchnic blood volume, and hepatic sulfobromophthalein clearance during general anesthesia in man. J Clin Invest 40:592–598
13. Mohamed MS, Bean JW (1951) Local and general alterations of blood CO_2 and influenceof intestinal motility in regulation of intestinal blood flow. Am J Physiol 167:413
14. Shimizu M, Hiroshi Y, Hatori N, Haga Y, Okuda E, Uriuda Y, Tanaka S (1990) Acute effect of intra-abdominal pressure on liver and systemic circulation. Vasc Surg 24:677–682
15. Caldwell CB, Ricotta JJ (1987) Changes in visceral blood flow with elevated intra-abdominal pressure. J Surg Res 43:14–20
16. Sala-Blanch X, Fontanals J, Delgado S, Martinez-Paiii G, Taura P, Lacy AM, Visa J (1996) Effects of carbon dioxide versus helium pneumoperitoneum on hepatic blood flow in pigs (abstract). Surg Endosc 10:183
17. Schein M, Wittmann DH, Aprahamian CC, Condon RE (1995) The abdominal compartment syndrome: the physiological and clinical consequences of elevated intra-abdominal pressure. J Am Col Surgeons 180:745–753
18. Harman PK, Kron IL, McLachlan HD et al (1982) Elevated intra-abdominal pressure and renal function. Ann Surg 196:594–597
19. Richards WO, Scovill W, Shin B, Reed W (1983) Acute renal failure associated with increased intra-abdominal pressure Ann Surg 197:183–187
20. Lieberman DA, Keefe EB, Rahatzad M, Keller FS (1983) Rupture abdominal aortic aneurysm causing obstructive jaundice. Dig Dis Sci 28:88–93
21. Savino JA, Cerabona T, Agarwal N, Byrne D (1988) Manipulation of ascitic fluid pressure in cirrhotics to optimize hemodynamic and renal function Ann Surg 253:504–510

6 Influence of Pneumoperitoneum on the Mesenteric Circulation

E. ELEFTHERIADIS and K. KOTZAMPASSI

Introduction

The technical advances of laparoscopic instrumentation and the impressive development of laparoscopic procedures in the last decade have been remarkable. But, as with all newly introduced surgical techniques, the initial swell of excitement is soon tempered by clinical reality.

The creation of pneumoperitoneum is a complex physiologic event, with attendant changes in the peritoneal environment and other homeostatic mechanisms. Although the physiologic systemic consequences of elevated intra-abdominal pressure (IAP) due to gas insufflation were recognized prior the introduction of laparoscopic cholecystectomy, only recently has it become apparent that pneumoperitoneum creates compartment syndrome with additional splanchnic disturbances.

Initially, in similar abdominal compartment syndromes occurring in a number of clinical situations, such as increased intraperitoneal or retroperitoneal bleeding, massive bowel distension due to mechanical obstruction or after hemorrhagic shock/resuscitation, intraperitoneal packing to control residual bleeding or tense ascites, one of the observed phenomena, insufficiently studied, was the finding of oliguria [22, 24]. Later, in the days of iatrogenic elevation of IAP for therapeutic purposes, it was discovered that oliguria originates during laparoscopic surgery due to decreased renal perfusion [5].

Studies performed on animals and adult humans dealing with the cardiovascular effects of peritoneal gas insufflation have shown physiologic derangement as a result of increased IAP. These systemic events seemed to be the cause of local compression on the parenchyma of the abdominal organs, but today an important factor in this situation is the aspect of reduced splanchnic perfusion [26].

Obviously, the visceral vascular bed is the primary site of this compression, and thus its collapse and that of the capillaries and small veins seems likely to decrease the perfusion in respective organs. This decrease in blood flow could result in deterioration of the organ's function, but to date the only clinical manifestation, as previously mentioned, arose in the kidney. Three main segments of the abdominal viscera could be influenced by raised IAP: the mesenteric, the liver, and the renal circulation.

This chapter describes the influence of increased IAP on the mesenteric blood flow and, consequently, on the gastrointestinal tract. The collected experimental and clinical data are presented and analyzed herein, but although the splanchnic vascular systems (as with all others) are functionally interactive and interdependent, we have tried to limit ourselves to mesenteric circulation. Additionally, the possible mechanisms involved in the changes in mesenteric circulation during increased IAP are discussed. Last but not least, the clinical significance of these data on laparoscopy patients is hypothesized.

Experimental Data

Over the last decade, several experimental investigations have indicated that increased IAP, independent of the technique used, has physiological effects on the abdominal viscera perfusion. A total of nine such studies have directly demonstrated that the mesenteric circulation is affected and that blood flow in the respective splanchnic organs is compromised (Table 1).

The first experimental evidence that the mesenteric circulation is influenced by increased IAP was presented by Barnes et al. [1] in 1985, the aim of their study being to determine the impact of elevated intraperitoneal hydrostatic pressure on the function of the cardiovascular system. The initial hypothesis of these investigators was as follows: since a number of clinical conditions are characterized by an excessive accumulation of fluid within the potential space of the peritoneal cavity, and as a direct consequence of this ascites-like formation there is an intraperitoneal pressure elevation, high pressure levels are likely to have an impact on the blood supply to the abdominal organs by reducing the effective perfusion pressure. In this study performed upon anesthetized dogs, the intra-abdominal fluid volume and hydrostatic pressure, from 0 to 40 mmHg, were step elevated by positive pressure infusion of Tyrode's solution into the peritoneal cavity, while blood flow in the celiac and superior mesenteric arteries was recorded by means of electromagnetic probes. It was found that increasing the IAP reduced the blood flow by 42% and 61%, respectively. The authors concluded that all of these reactions are graded in accordance with the degree of intraperitoneal hypertension. When the pressure level is below 20 mmHg, the effects are mild, but at higher pressures, the severity of the detrimental reactions increases dramatically.

Two years later, in 1987, Caldwell and Ricotta [4], in an effort to quantify the changes in visceral blood flow after IAP elevation, measured the blood flow of all abdominal organs (stomach, duodenum, jejunum, ileum, colon, pancreas, liver, spleen, kidney and adrenal glands) in dogs. An inflatable bag was placed intra-abdominally to create graded increases of IAP, and visceral blood flow was assessed at baseline and at 20 and 40 mmHg by using the radioactive microspheres technique. The organ blood flow index (OBFI) was then determined for each organ by the use of the formula (OBFI=OBF/cardiac output). Elevated IAP was found to cause a decrease in the absolute blood flow for all organs measured, except the adrenal glands where the blood flow was increased. Similarly, the OBFI was decreased significantly for all intra-abdominal viscera, except the renal cortex and the adrenal glands. The authors concluded that the changes in organ blood flow are more marked than can be accounted for by changes in cardiac output alone, suggesting that local control mechanisms may be responsible for changes in visceral blood flow. However, the data of this experiment raise, for

Table 1. Experimental data on intra-abdominal pressure and mesenteric circulation

	SMABF	Splanchnic micro-circulation	PVF	PVP	Intestinal micro-circulation	Intestinal pHi mucosal	Intestinal O_2 extraction	Splanchnic free radicals	Bacterial trans-location
Barnes, 1985 [1]	↓								
Caldwell, 1987 [4]		↓							
Shimizu, 1990 [27]			↓	↑					
Diebel, 1992 [6]	↓				↓	↓			
Diebel, 1992 [7]			↓						
Kotzampassi, 1993 [17]				↑	↓	↓			
Ishizaki, 1993 [13]	↓		↓						
Ischizaki, 1993 [14]	↓		↓						
Eleftheriadis, 1996 [9]					↓		↓	↑	↑

SMABF, superior mesenteric artery blood flow;
PVF, portal vein flow;
PVP, portal vein pressure.

the first time, the possibility that IAP elevation could be of clinical significance, since such decreases in blood flow may result in splanchnic ischemia and organ dysfunction or failure, if the increase in pressure is severe enough. On the other hand, one could note that, although this paper was published in the year the first laparoscopic cholecystectomy was performed, the investigative interest of the authors was directed towards the splanchnic consequences of raised IAP from causes other than the artificially created pneumoperitoneum, i.e., from tense ascites, intra-abdominal bleeding, or after application of anti-shock trousers.

In 1990, Shimizu et al. [27] attempted to study the acute effects of IAP – due to intraperitoneal or retroperitoneal bleeding after abdominal trauma or following surgery – on liver and systemic circulation. The portal vein blood flow (measured by means of an electromagnetic flowmeter) and the portal vein pressure were measured in dogs at IAP levels of 10–40 mmHg achieved by colloid solution infusion into the abdominal cavity. They found that IAP had a good correlation with portal vein pressure, but an inverse relation to portal vein blood flow. Since the results of this investigation indicate that portal hemodynamics are affected by the elevation of IAP, the authors suggested that the increased pressure has a negative influence on liver function. Additionally, the parallel increase found in femoral vein pressure lead them to the opinion that all intra-abdominal organs are affected by afterload. But considering that portal circulation comprises the upstream part of mesenteric circulation, one can deduce that the downstream part would also be affected by IAP.

In 1992, Diebel et al. [6] published the results of their study on the macro- and microcirculatory effects of increased intraperitoneal pressure on intestinal blood flow in anesthetized pigs. Superior mesenteric artery blood flow, intestinal mucosal microcirculation and gastric intramucosal pH (pHi) measured by means of ultrasonic transit-time technique, laser Doppler flowmetry, and tonometry, respectively, were evaluated as IAP was raised to 10, 20, 30, and 40 mmHg by infusing lactated Ringer's solution intraperitoneally. A 20-mmHg pressure was found causing significant decreases both in mesenteric artery blood flow and intestinal mucosal microcirculation, the changes becoming progressively greater as the hydrostatic pressure was increased to 40 mmHg. At this level the pHi fell to 6.98, indicating severe mucosal ischemia. The profound decreases in mucosal and mesenteric blood flow were reversed upon gradual release of IAP by evacuating the crystalloid solution instilled into the peritoneal cavity. The results of this study clearly show that there was a severe progressive decrease in splanchnic hemodynamics at an IAP of 20 mmHg or higher, thus giving a complete answer to what happens to mesenteric circulation when the intraperitoneal pressure increases dramatically during massive bowel distention or intra/retroperitoneal bleeding. Although these changes were observed at pressures much above those used for laparoscopic surgery, Diebel et al. [6] registered a decrease in intestinal mucosal microcirculation to 81% of the baseline measurement, at a pressure of 10 mmHg. However, the major import of this experiment is the detection for the first time, by means of tonometry, of intestinal ischemia caused by increased IAP, although this speculation had previously been made by other investigators [4].

Simultaneously with the previous paper, Diebel and coworkers [7] published another experimental study on the same animal model, dealing with the effects of increased IAP on hepatic artery and portal vein blood flow, assessed by the ultrasonic transit-time technique, as well as on hepatic microcirculation. Although cardiac output and mean arterial pressure were at normal levels, portal vein blood flow fell significantly by 27% of the control value at 10 mmHg IAP, and by 65% at 20 mmHg IAP. The results of this study, reproducing those of Shimizu et al. [27], clearly indicate that not only a modest increase in IAP causes significant impairment of hepatic perfusion, but that severe hemodynamic disturbances also occur in the out-flow of mesenteric circulation.

Up until 1992 the efforts of all investigators to study the effects of increased intraperitoneal pressure on splanchnic viscera were based on the creation of tense hydroperitoneum or inflation of an intra-abdominally positioned bag. That was a realistic animal model for the study of some clinical situations, but laparoscopic surgery with gas insufflation was already 6 years old. Therefore, hydroperitoneum had to be replaced by pneumoperitoneum induced by CO_2 insufflation, and the intraperitoneal pressures had to be reduced to 15 mmHg.

In 1993, Kotzampassi et al. [17] published the hemodynamic effects occurring in the peritoneal environment during pneumoperitoneum in dogs. In this experiment, the intestinal mucosa microcirculation and the intestinal mucosa pHi assessed by means of laser Doppler flowmetry and tonometry, respectively, as well as the portal pressure, were studied at 14 mmHg IAP, in baseline conditions and 1, 2, 5, 15, 30, 45, and 60 min thereafter. Portal pressure had a threefold increase which diminished rapidly after peritoneal cavity deflation at the end of the experiment. This result is in agreement with the finding of Shimizu et al. [27]. Intestinal mucosal microcirculation was reduced after increasing IAP to 50% of the baseline value within 5 min, and remained constant throughout the experiment. This finding of tissue hypoperfusion was further documented by the tonometric catheter which revealed, at the end of the experiment, a reduction of intestinal mucosa pHi to 6.80. Such a value is so much lower than the normal value and, as the above findings reconfirm the results of Diebel et al. [6], the conclusion of splanchnic ischemia is inescapable. However, this raises the question of whether bacterial translocation can be provoked and to what degree these findings hold true for human beings.

Another paper dealing with changes in splanchnic blood flow and cardiovascular effects following peritoneal insufflation was published by Ishizaki et al. [13]. Superior mesenteric artery and portal vein blood flow, using the ultrasonic transit-time technique, were measured in dogs at an intraperitoneal pressure of 16 mmHg during a 3-h period. They found that blood flow in both vessels was decreased as early as 30 min after starting insufflation, with the decline persisting throughout the course of pneumoperitoneum. A version of this study, published by Ishizaki et al. [13] in the same year, reports similar findings related to the superior mesenteric artery and portal vein blood flow. The results of these two studies are in agreement with the findings of other investigators using the same techniques [1, 6, 7, 27], and reconfirm that impairment of mesenteric circulation during IAP elevation is a fact.

All the above-mentioned experimental studies lead to the conclusion that mesenteric ischemia exists during intraperitoneal pressure elevation. However, it is well known that mild, moderate, or severe splanchnic ischemia of either etiology may facilitate bacterial translocation through a number of different mechanisms that depend on both the degree and duration of ischemia [32]. On the other hand, increased IAP after gas insufflation for laparoscopic surgery, and subsequent decreased IAP after deflation at the end of the operation, could be considered to be a complete mechanism producing intestinal ischemia/ reperfusion. Haglund [10] claims that the reperfusion component of ischemic injury is more pronounced after partial than after total ischemia; therefore, further studies dealing with the splanchnic influence of tense pneumoperitoneum should be undertaken.

During 1996, Eleftheriadis et al. [9], investigated experimentally whether tension pneumoperitoneum leads to intestinal ischemia and, as a consequence, to the production of free radicals and bacterial translocation. The following parameters were measured in rats subjected to a 15-mmHg pressure insufflation for 60 min: the intestinal mucosal microcirculation (by means of laser Doppler flowmetry), the gut metabolic activity (O_2 extraction, by blood sampling from portal vein/carotid artery), the intestinal, hepatic, splenic, and lung free radical production (malondialdehyde), and the bacterial translocation toward the mesenteric lymph nodes, liver, and spleen, at 3 h and 18 h after pneumoperitoneum deflation. Intestinal mucosal microcirculation was significantly decreased, as was the gut metabolic activity, while the malondialdehyde levels, indicators of free radical production, were found to be increased in all studied organs 30 min after abdominal deflation. Finally, bacterial translocation toward the mesenteric lymph nodes, spleen, and liver was increased in the 3-h group; in the 18-h group bacteria were not found in the mesenteric lymph nodes, but were in the liver and spleen. The authors concluded that, although these findings are impressive, they must be reproduced in humans and their clinical significance clarified. This paper confirms the results of previous studies [4, 6, 17] that the intestinal mucosa microcirculation is compromised during IAP elevation, but the new knowledge arising from this investigation is that pneumoperitoneum leads to gut metabolic activity impairment, results in ischemia/reperfusion injury to various organs, and creates bacterial translocation.

Clinical Data

Although the hemodynamic effects of peritoneal insufflation on the cardiovascular and pulmonary systems have been widely studied in laparoscopic surgery patients [23], its effects on human splanchnic perfusion have not been determined. The results of the previously-mentioned experimental studies are difficult to reproduce in humans for methodological and ethical reasons and because such research must be performed under strictly monitored conditions. Two clinical studies have investigated the possible relationship between abnormally low pHi readings and increased IAP due to causes other than gas insufflation. Another three clinical studies have attempted to prove the existence of splanchnic ischemia during laparoscopic surgery by means of the non-invasive techniques of laser Doppler flowmetry and tonometry (Table 2).

Table 2. Clinical data on intra-abdominal pressure and mesenteric circulation

	Gastric pHi	Splanchnic microcirculation
Pusajo, 1994 [21]	↓	
Eleftheriadis, 1996 [8]	↓	↓
Thaler, 1996 [29]	—	
Benecke, 1996 [3]		↓
Sugrue, 1996 [28]	↓	
Windsor, 1996 [33]	↓	

pHi, gastric intramucosal pH.

Pusajo et al. [21] were probably the first to refer to a correlation between intraperitoneal pressure and pHi existence after their studies of ten patients with increased IAP (10 mmHg), from causes other than gas insufflation.

In 1996, Eleftheriadis et al. [8] measured the gastric mucosal pHi by means of a tonometric nasogastric catheter during peritoneal insufflation at a constant pressure of 12 mmHg, and after abdominal deflation, in eight laparoscopic cholecystectomy patients; an equal number of open cholecystectomy patients served as controls. Gastric pHi was found significantly decreased in laparoscopic surgery patients in relation to controls (7.15 vs. 7.37), while gastric pHi returned to its normal values (7.15 vs. 7.43) immediately after abdominal deflation. The results of this clinical investigation are the first reproduction in laparoscopic patients of the experimentally proven and tonometrically detected splanchnic ischemia during elevation of IAP [6, 17].

Shortly thereafter, Thaler et al. [29] published a similarly designed clinical investigation where the gastric mucosal pHi was also recorded tonometrically. They found that, in spite of increased IAP, no decrease in pHi was registered during laparoscopic surgery and, therefore, the evidence of splanchnic ischemia was not prominent.

Since the results of these two studies conflict, an explanation must be attempted. Bearing in mind that it is currently accepted that acid secretion inhibition is mandatory for proper assessment of gastric mucosal pHi [16], the lack of information in the study of Eleftheriadis et al. [8] of such pharmaceutical manipulation could lead to the suggestion that the authors overestimated the gastric pHi. However, the preoperative administration of a proton pump inhibitor is in routine use at their anesthesia department. On the other hand, in this study, the decreased hepatic microcirculation documented by the percutaneously positioned laser Doppler fiber could be considered as a fact of splanchnic hypoperfusion. However, the existence or the absence of low gastric mucosal pHi in laparoscopic surgery patients needs further confirmation.

According to recent information arising from Windsor [33], Bonham et al. demonstrated significant gastric mucosal ischemia, with intra-abdominal pressures of more than 8 mmHg, by using a nasogastric tonometer in patients undergoing laparoscopic cholecystectomy.

In 1996, Benecke et al. [3] performed a clinical study, published in abstract form, dealing with the microcirculatory changes of all intra-abdominal organs during laparoscopy. The microcirculation in the gastric wall, the duodenum, jejunum, colon, and liver, as well as in the parietal peritoneum and abdominal wall, were measured by means of laser Doppler flowmetry at an IAP of 0, 10, and 14 mmHg. The elevation of IAP from 0 to 14 mmHg, but not from 0 to 10 mmHg, significantly decreases the microcirculation in the abdominal wall and parietal peritoneum, as well as in the gastric wall, while it was found to decrease, although not significantly, in the duodenum, jejunum, colon, and liver. Furthermore, the decrease of blood flow correlated significantly with the operation time. The results of this study reproduce those of other investigators using the laser Doppler technique [6, 8, 9, 17] and adds the information that these changes are also time dependent.

Finally, in the same year, Sugrue et al. [28] made an effort to study the potential association between postoperatively increased IAP by measuring bladder pressure and abnormally low gastric intramucosal pHi by means of gastric tonometry. Measurements were made three times daily in 73 intensive care patients undergoing major abdominal open surgery. Considering abnormal pressures to be equal or more than 20 mmHg and pHi equal or less than 7.32, they concluded that there is a significant association between increased IAP and pHi.

Conclusions

Much of the pathophysiology associated with laparoscopy was rediscovered in the years following the first laparoscopic cholecystectomy. The regional (intra-abdominal) influences of raised intraperitoneal pressure, with special interest in mesenteric hemodynamics, have been investigated over the last 11 years, leading to the publication of nine experimental and five clinical studies. There is a growing understanding that elevated IAP, of whatever etiology, creates a compartment syndrome exhibiting severe disturbances to mesenteric circulation and placing all intra-abdominal viscera under ischemic conditions. It is of interest that the level of pressure needed for the appearance of splanchnic hemodynamic alterations is about 15 mmHg, a pressure normally used for laparoscopic surgery.

Several mechanisms are considered to be implicated in the decrease in splanchnic blood flow due to elevated IAP: Increased IAP has a direct influence, by means of mechanical compression, on abdominal arteries, veins, and visceral organs, as well as on the abdominal wall surfaces. As the diaphragm is pushed upward the thoracic cavity is also compressed, thus raising intrathoracic pressure and leading to the compression of heart, lungs, and major vessels within the thoracic cavity [2]. Since the trunks of major vessels are located within the thoracic and peritoneal cavities, it seems logical that high pressure exerted on them will be transmitted indirectly to the distant organs perfused [1]. Thus, the initial increase of IAP elicits a chain of mechanical reactions which affect macro- and microcirculation.

In all the studies mentioned, both experimental and clinical, the main effect of raised IAP, due to either etiology, was the blood flow reduction in the superior mesenteric artery [6]. However, according to Caldwell and Ricotta [4] decreases seen in abdominal visceral blood flow apart from that of the adrenal glands, are greater than those which could be accounted for by the alteration (decrease) in cardiac output. Considering that the pressure gradient-driving flow is calculated by the difference between systemic arterial pressure and intraperitoneal pressure, it is probable that an increase in IAP would lead to vascular resistance elevation. Mechanisms for this increase in systemic vascular resistance have not been fully elucidated up to now, but are probably due primary to the mechanical compression of the splanchnic capillary beds and the subsequent rise in splanchnic vascular resistance caused by the elevated IAP [2, 4, 13]. The increased vascular resistance leads to a consequent vasoconstriction which may be affected by neural, hormonal, or intrinsic influences: Increased partial CO_2 pressure in blood due to CO_2 absorption [9, 12] after pneumoperitoneum induction, accounts for an increased, hypercapnia-induced sympathicotonia which causes peripheral and mesenteric vasoconstriction [13, 26]. It is of interest to note that after helium, argon, or nitric oxide insufflation, neither arterial blood pressure increased nor hypercapnia occurred [18, 19].

Arterial hypoxemia due to high IAP may contribute to vasoconstriction. Although increased levels of arterial PCO_2 have been shown to have a positive inotropic effect on the myocardium which influences cardiac output and systemic vascular resistance [34], it is believed that hemodynamic disturbances during laparoscopic surgery are mainly attributable to the decreased venous return [1, 31].

Decreased transcardial pressures may elicit a reflex vasoconstriction through the atrial receptors, while the reduced stretch of these receptors may also cause vasopressin release which is widely accepted as a vasoconstrictor of splanchnic vasculature [1].

Liberation of systemically active vasoconstrictors like vasopressin from the gut have been considered to be the cause of reduced blood flow from the mesenteric, renal, and celiac vasculature [20] during laparoscopy [13, 26], while Husain et al. [12] suggest that vasopressin is released by peripheral pain receptor activation in the case of abdominal wall distention by pneumoperitoneum. Additionally, reduced renal perfusion due to kidney compression leads to angiotensin release [25].

Concerning the venous system, increased IAP exhibits a direct mechanical effect, i.e., the collapse of splanchnic veins and thus the decrease of venous backflow and the increase of preload [26]. Since Poiseuille's law states that the blood flow in a vessel is proportional to the fourth power of its radius, even a small decrease in blood vessel diameter leads to a significant decrease of blood flow and extreme vascular resistance elevation [13]. In particular, compression of the portal vein, which represents the major outflow tract of mesenteric circulation, leads to blood flow stasis and intravascular pressure elevation, and thereby triggers an intrinsic myogenically mediated vasoconstriction [1]. The decreased gut mucosal perfusion, as assessed by laser Doppler flowmetry [3, 6, 17] seems to be the consequence of the increased portal pressure. Similar findings are reported by Kiel et al. [15], who found a significant reduction in total and mucosal microcirculation after venous outflow pressure elevation in a chambered canine stomach preparation.

On the other hand, since visceral organ surfaces are also compressed by the increased IAP, the extravascular pressure is probably elevated, a response that would tend towards a reduction of vessel distention and to a myogenic vasodilation acceleration, since it is accepted that a well developed myogenic mechanism for the local control of the vascular tone exists [13].

Additionally, a high IAP is likely to have a direct impact on the blood supply of the abdominal organs by reducing effective perfusion pressures. It seems likely that the capillaries and small veins would collapse, thus decreasing circulation to the viscera and causing stasis and fluid exudation [14]. Shimizu [27] supports the opinion of a direct mechanical effect, based on the fact that the parallel increase of femoral vein pressure and IAP suggest that all intravisceral organs are affected by afterload [11].

The mortality rate associated with laparoscopic cholecystectomy is generally agreed to be low [30]. Clinical practice has shown patients to have an uneventful postoperative course and none of the complications discussed herein appears to have occurred. As surgeons have become increasingly comfortable with the use of the laparoscope it seems logical to attempt more complex procedures of longer duration under raised IAP. Therefore, we would expect the splanchnic ischemia to be prolonged and thus its effect on abdominal viscera, healthy or dysfunctional, to be unknown.

Recent improvement in the knowledge of reperfusion injury lead us to assess all events in the light of free radical-induced damage, since abdominal deflation following a laparoscopic procedure is an example of such a reperfusion injury of previously poorly perfused organs. These results, although difficult to reproduce in humans, raise questions as to the possibility of bacterial translocation and septic complications in immunocompromised patients or patients suffering immunological deficiency. Additionally, with the rapid expansion of laparoscopic surgery, patient demographics have shifted and more elderly individuals, often at higher operative risk, are undergoing increasingly lengthy laparoscopic surgical procedures.

The above experimental and clinical data lead us to conclude that elevated intraperitoneal pressure, including the etiology of gas insufflation, decreases mesenteric circulation and produces splanchnic organ ischemia. The clinical significance of these findings is unknown and remains to be clarified by well designed studies.

Summary

Abdominal insufflation for laparoscopic procedures leads to numerous hemodynamic effects. Besides peripheral vascular and central cardiopulmonary

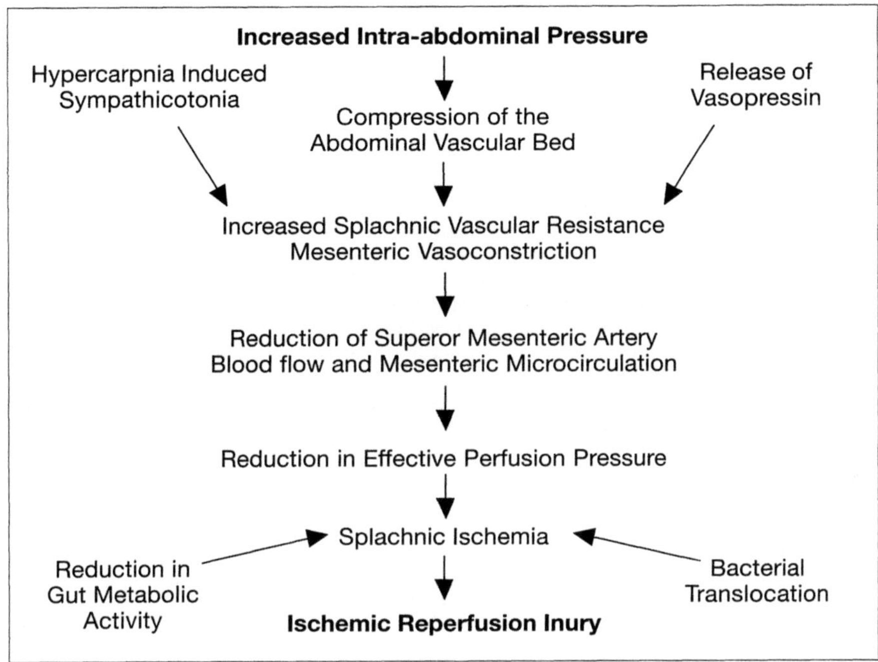

Fig. 1. Hemodynamic effects of abdominal insufflation for laparoscopic procedures

changes during pneumoperitoneum, splanchnic perfusion is most affected. Experimental studies have shown that the superior mesenteric artery blood flow, the intestinal mucosal microcirculation, and intramucosal pHi are reduced. In addition, the portal blood flow decreases, while the portal blood pressure increases. Consequences of these changes are that the splanchnic production of free radicals increases, gut metabolic activity decreases, and bacterial translocation occurs (Fig. 1). Clinical studies performed on laparoscopic cholecystectomy patients have shown that, during gas insufflation, the gastric mucosal pHi is decreased, as well as the microcirculation of various abdominal viscera. The general impression from these data is that during laparoscopic surgery the abdominal organs are hypoperfused, but the clinical significance of this event needs to be investigated.

References

1. Barnes GE, Laine GA, Giam PY, Smith EE, Granger HJ (1985) Cardiovascular responses to elevation of intraabdominal hydrostatic pressure. Am J Physiol 248:R208
2. Baxter JN, O'Dwyer PJ (1995) Pathophysiology of laparoscopy. Br J Surg 82:1–2
3. Benecke P, Schiedeck T, Vatankhah M, Bruck HF (1996) Microcirculatory changes in intraabdominal organs depend on intraaabdominal pressure and operation time. Surg Endosc 5:546

4. Caldwell CB, Ricotta JJ (1987) Changes in visceral blood flow with elevated intraabdominal pressure. J Surg Res 43:14–20
5. Chiu AW, Chang LS, Birkett DH, Babayan RK (1995) The impact of pneumoperitoneum, pneumoretroperitoneum, and gasless laparoscopy on the systemic and renal hemodynamics. J Am Coll Surg 181:397–406
6. Diebel LN, Dulchavsky SA, Wilson RF (1992) Effect of increased intraabdominal pressure on mesenteric arterial and intestinal mucosal blood flow. J Trauma 33:45–49
7. Diebel WN, Wilson RF, Dulchavsky SA, Saxe J (1992) Effect of increased intraabdominal pressure on hepatic arterial, portal venous, and hepatic microcirculatory blood flow. J Trauma 33:279–283
8. Eleftheriadis E, Kotzampassi K, Botsios D, Tzartinoglou E, Farmakis H, Dadoukis J (1996) Splanchnic ischemia during laparoscopic cholecystectomy. Surg Endosc 10:324–326
9. Eleftheriadis E, Kotzampassi K, Papanotas K, Heliadis N, Sarris K (1996) Gut ischemia, oxidative stress, and bacterial translocation in elevated abdominal pressure in rats. World J Surg 20:11–16
10. Haglund UH (1994) Gut ischemia. Gut 35 [Suppl 1]:S73–S76
11. Hunter JG (1995) Laparoscopic pneumoperitoneum: the abdominal compartment syndrome revisited. J Am Coll Surg 181:469–470
12. Husain MK, Manger WM, Rock TW (1979) Vasopressin release due to manual restraint in the rat: role of body compression with other stressful stimuli. Endocrinology 10:641–644
13. Ishizaki Y, Bandai Y, Shimomura K, Abe H, Ohtomo Y, Idezuki Y (1993) Changes in splanchnic blood flow and cardiovascular effects following peritoneal insufflation of carbon dioxide. Surg Endosc 7:420–423
14. Ishizaki Y, Bandai Y, Shimomura K, Abe H, Ohtomo Y, Idezuki Y (1993) Safe intraabdominal pressure of carbon dioxide pneumoperitoneum during laparoscopic surgery. Surgery 114:549–554
15. Kiel JW, Riedel GL, Shepherd AP (1988) Metabolic and myogenic control of gastric mucosal blood flow. In: Manabe H, Zweifach BW, Messmer K (eds) Microcirculation in circulatory disorders. Springer, Tokyo, pp 195–204
16. Kolkman J, Groeneveld A, Meuwissen S (1994) Effect of ranitidine on basal and bicarbonate enhanced intragastric pCO_2: a tonometric study. Gut 35:737–741
17. Kotzampassi K, Kapanidis N, Kazamias P, Eleftheriadis E (1993) Hemodynamic events in the peritoneal environment during pneumoperitoneum in dogs. Surg Endosc 7:494–499
18. Leighton TA, Liu SY, Bongard FS (1993) Comparative cardiopulmonary effects of carbon dioxide versus helium pneumoperitoneum. Surgery 113:527–531
19. Phillips RS, Goldberg RI, Watson PW, Marshall JR, Barkin JS (1987) Mechanism of improved patient tolerance to nitrous oxide in diagnostic laparoscopy. Am J Gastroenterol 82:143–144
20. Punnonen R, Viinamaki O (1982) Vasopressin release during laparoscopy: role of increased intraabdominal pressure. Lancet i:175–176
21. Pusajo J, Bumaschny E, Agurrola A et al (1994) Postoperative intraabdominal pressure: its relation to splanchnic perfusion, sepsis, multiple organ failure and surgical reintervention. Int Crit Care Dig 13:2
22. Richards WO, Scovill W, Shin B, Reed W (1983) Acute renal failure associated with increased intraabdominal pressure. Ann Surg 197:183–187
23. Safran DB, Orlando R (1994) Physiologic effects of pneumoperitoneum. Am J Surg 167:281–286
24. Savino JA, Cerabona T, Agarwal N, Byrne D (1988) Manipulation of ascitic fluid pressure in cirrhotics to optimize hemodynamic and renal function. Ann Surg 208:504–511
25. Saxe JM, Ledgerwood AM, Lucas CE (1993) Management of the difficult abdominal closure. Surg Clin N Am 73:243–251
26. Schilling M, Krähenbühl L, Friess H, Zgraggen K, Büchler MW (1996) Physiological changes during pneumoperitoneum. Dig Surg 13:2–5
27. Shimizu M, Yohizu H, Hatori N, Haga Y, Okuda E, Uriuda Y, Tanaka S (1990) Acute effect of intraabdominal pressure on liver and systemic circulation. Vasc Surg 24:677–682
28. Sugrue M, Jones F, Lee A, Buist MD, Deane S, Bauman A, Hillman K (1996) Intraabdominal pressure and gastric intramucosal pH: is there an association? World J Surg 20:988–991
29. Thaler W, Frey L, Marzoli GP, Messmer K (1996) Assessment of splanchnic tissue oxygenation by gastric tonometry in patients undergoing laparoscopic and open cholecystectomy. Br J Surg 83:620–624

30. The Southern Surgeons Club (1991) A prospective analysis of 1518 laparoscopic cholecystectomies. N Engl J Med 324:1073–1078
31. Torrielli R, Cesarini M, Winnock S, Cabiro C, Mene JM (1990) Modifications hemodynamiques durant la coelioscopie: étude menée par bio impédance électrique thoracique. Can J Anaesth 37:1, 46–51
32. Wells CL, Maddaus MA, Simmons RL (1989) Bacterial translocation. In: Marston A, Bulkley GB, Fiddian-Green RO, Haglund UH (eds) Splanchnic ischemia and multiple organ failure. Edward Arnold, London, pp 195–204
33. Windsor JA (1996) Invited commentary to the paper: Gut ischemia, oxidative stress, and bacterial translocation in elevated abdominal pressure in rats, by Eleftheriadis E et al. World J Surg 20:11–16
34. Wittgen CM, Andrus CH, Fitzgerald SD, Bandendistel LJ, Dahms TE, Kaminski DL (1991) Analysis of the hemodynamic and ventilatory effects of laparoscopic cholecystectomy. Arch Surg 126:997–1001

7 Renal Function and Circulation Under the Influence of Pneumoperitoneum

L.N. Diebel

Introduction

In 1923*, Thorington and Schmidt [1] were stimulated to investigate the effects of increased intra-abdominal pressure (IAP) on renal function in a patient with malignant ascites whose urine output improved following paracentesis. In a subsequent canine study they demonstrated that the animals became oliguric at an IAP of 15–30 mmHg and anuric when IAP exceeded 30 mmHg.

In recent years, a number of clinical situations involving acutely increased IAP have been causally related to subsequent renal impairment. These include the following:
- Postoperative or post-traumatic intra-abdominal or retroperitoneal bleeding
- Post-resuscitation visceral edema
- Bowel obstruction or ileus
- Abdominal packing
- Inflammatory conditions such as diffuse peritonitis or hemorrhagic pancreatitis
- Pneumatic anti-shock garment
- Laparoscopic procedures

This chapter concerns in particular the cardiovascular effects of pneumoperitoneum used for laparoscopic procedures. Following initial experience with laparoscopic cholecystectomies, the laparoscopic technique has been employed as an effective alternative to standard surgical approaches in the treatment of a variety of operable diseases. Procedures such as fundoplication, lymphadenectomy, vagotomy/gastrectomy, and colonic resection are now being performed laparoscopically. Obviously, these increasingly complex procedures often require lengthy operating times. Thus, there is heightened concern about the effects of IAP from the CO_2 pneumoperitoneum on the systemic circulation and the various intra-abdominal organs.

This chapter reviews basic renal physiology and published information on renal hemodynamics and function with increased IAP.

Review of Normal Renal Physiology

Under normal circumstances the kidneys receive 20%–25% (1.25 l/min) of the cardiac output. Most (85%) of the renal blood flow (RBF) perfuses the outer cortex of the kidney. The remaining 15% of RBF perfuses the juxtamedullary nephrons. Blood flow to the kidneys is determined by cardiac output and renal vascular resistance. RBF is maintained relatively constant, despite significant changes in mean arterial pressure, by autoregulatory resistance changes in the renal afferent arteriole.

Approximately 20% of the renal plasma flow (650 ml/min) is filtered as an essentially protein-free plasma through the glomerular capillary into Bowman's capsule. This glomerular filtration process is governed by Starling forces and averages 125 ml/min or 180 l/day (glomerular filtration rate, GFR).

A number of hormones and mediators help regulate renal function. Among these different hormones prostaglandins appear to have a central role [2]. Prostaglandins are probably responsible for the release of renin from the juxtaglomerular apparatus (JGA). Renin is also released in response to decreased renal perfusion pressure, renal sympathetic stimulation, and reduced sodium delivery to the JGA. Circulating renin cleaves an a_2-globulin to produce angiotensin I, a weak vasoconstrictor, which converts to angiotensin II, a potent vasoconstrictor.

Other important hormones controlling various aspects of renal function include aldosterone and antidiuretic hormone (ADH). Aldosterone stimulates sodium reabsorption primarily in the distal tubules and collecting ducts. Secretion of aldosterone is controlled by plasma sodium and potassium concentrations, adrenocorticotropic hormone (ACTH), and angiotensin. ADH released under the control of baroreceptors and osmoreceptors leads to increased permeability of the collecting ducts to water, net water reabsorption, and increased urine osmolarity.

Recently, the L-arginine–nitric oxide (NO) pathway has been shown to play an important role in the control of various renal functions [3]. NO is known to regulate several physiologic renal processes, including intrarenal blood flow, ultrafiltration, and sodium excretion. Although a role for the renin-angiotensin axis, and aldosterone and ADH secretion is suggested in the renal response to increased IAP (see below), a role for prostaglandins or nitric oxide remains speculative.

Experimental Studies Relating to Intra-abdominal Pressure and Renal Function

A number of experimental models have been used to study the hemodynamic effects of increased IAP. Generalizations based on these studies concerning the renal effects of increased IAP are somewhat confounded because of several variables in the methodologies used:
- Species of animal and type of anesthesia used
- Method used to increase IAP and level of IAP attained
- Method or methods used to attempt to control the effects of IAP on cardiac output when assessing renal hemodynamic effects
- Methods used to assess renal hemodynamics and function
- Assessment of renal and central hemodynamic effects when IAP returns to baseline

The importance of controlling these variables is best exemplified by changes in cardiac output with IAP. Cardiac output may decrease with increasing IAP and thus by itself negatively impact RBF. It is difficult, therefore, to discern the direct effect of IAP on renal hemodynamics and function under these circumstances.

Caldwell and Ricotta [4] used an inflatable bag placed intra-abdominally in nine dogs to create graded increases in IAP. Hemodynamic parameters and organ blood flow obtained using radioactive microspheres were measured at baseline and after increasing IAP to 20 and 40 mmHg. Visceral blood flow decreased to all intra-abdominal organs with the exception of the adrenal gland. Because cardiac output was significantly depressed at both 20 and 40 mg Hg IAP organ blood flow was indexed to cardiac output (organ blood flow index, OBFI). Of note, the gastrointestinal viscera showed a significant fall in the OBFI with elevated IAP. The OBFI for the renal cortex was essentially unchanged, indicating that the decreases in renal cortical blood flow could be accounted for by the alterations in cardiac output. The effects of increasing cardiac output to baseline values or abdominal decompression on visceral blood flow were not assessed in this study.

In another canine model of increased IAP, Barnes et al. [5] reported a 36% reduction in cardiac output and stroke volume after IAP was increased to 40 mmHg by the intraperitoneal infusion of an isotonic solution. Flow in the celiac, superior mesenteric, and renal arteries was reduced by 42%, 61%, and 70%, respectively. Resistance changes were calculated to increase by 26% in the celiac artery, 90% in the superior mesenteric, and 136% in the renal artery. Of particular note in this study is the variable changes in visceral blood flow and vascular resistance in the different splanchnic beds reported.

Harman et al. [6] investigated the relative effect of increased IAP on cardiac output and renal function in another canine model. RBF and GFR were derived from para-aminohippurate (PAH) and inulin clearances, respectively. Hemodynamic and renal function measurements were made at baseline, 20, and 40 mgHg IAP. RBF and GFR decreased to about 22% of baseline when IAP was 20 mmHg. Cardiac output was reduced to only 79% of baseline at this level of IAP. At 40 mmHg IAP three of seven dogs became anuric, and the RBF and GFR of the remaining dogs was 6%–7% of baseline, while cardiac output was reduced to 37% of baseline. The animals were then volume expanded with a colloid infusion. Although cardiac output was pushed to 200% of baseline, RBF and GFR remained at 20% of baseline in the volume expanded animals at 40 mmHg IAP.

Subsequent abdominal decompression led to a further increase in cardiac output. RBF and GFR approached but did not reach baseline values 30 min after abdominal decompression. Renal vascular resistance was markedly elevated at both 20 and 40 mmHg IAP. A possible role of ureteral compression on renal hemodynamics and function was eliminated in two animals by the placement of ureteral stents.

Chiu et al. [7] used a porcine model to study the renal hemodynamic effects of CO_2 pneumoperitoneum. This model is clinically relevant to laparoscopic procedures because CO_2 pneumoperitoneum was used to increase IAP to 15 mmHg. Renal cortical tissue perfusion was assessed using laser Doppler flowmetry at baseline and 15 mmHg IAP. The renal tissue perfusion was 50 ± 18 ml/min per

100 g tissue during the preinsufflation phase, and it decreased to 20 ± 5 ml/100 g tissue when IAP reached 15 mmHg. The persistent decrease in renal cortical tissue perfusion during pneumoperitoneum returned immediately to the preinsufflation level once the pressure was released.

From these animal studies, it is apparent that the adverse effects of IAP on renal hemodynamics are due to changes in cardiac output and a direct effect on RBF. As noted, Harman et al. [6] demonstrated that the renal perfusion deficit with increased IAP persists despite normal or even supranormal values of cardiac output. Thus changes in renal vascular resistance, the other determinant of RBF, are critical in the understanding of the pathophysiology of increased IAP on renal function.

A number of factors may act to increase renal vascular resistance with increased IAP:

- The role of ureteral compression for the decreased urine output noted with increased IAP has been discounted by experimental and clinical reports [6]. In these studies ureteral stents were placed and failed to resolve the impaired renal function observed with increased IAP. This is consistent with the observation by Vaughan et al. [8] that with acute ureteral obstruction, the renal collecting system can generate pressures up to 90 mmHg. Vaughan also demonstrated that RBF increases acutely with ureteral obstruction, contrary to what has been reported with increased IAP. Next, direct renal compression has been shown to elevate cortical pressures, placing the renal parenchyma at risk of ischemia and causing a so called "renal compartment syndrome" [9]. It has been postulated that this may occur with increased IAP.
- Renal venous pressure changes closely mimic the increases in IAP [6, 10]. The resultant renal venous hypertension may increase renal vascular resistance by mechanically obstructing renal venous outflow and leading to a secondary decrease in renal artery blood flow.
- The renal vasoconstrictor effects may be due to neural or hormonal influences. Increased sympathetic activity may occur from the elevated IAP or from arterial hypercarbia [11, 12]. Arterial hypercarbia may occur due to hypoventilation or from absorbed CO_2 used to create the pneumoperitoneum.
- Hormonal changes with IAP were first reported by Le Roith and colleagues [13]. They demonstrated that abdominal pressure (80 mmHg) caused an elevation of plasma ADH to more than twice basal levels. Prior infusion of dextran prevented this elevation of ADH levels and the associated 20% fall in cardiac output with the increased IAP. Presumably the increased plasma ADH levels were mediated by activation of central baroreceptors.
- More recently, Bloomfield et al. [10] measured the plasma renin activity (PRA), aldosterone, and atrial natriuretic factor (ANF) responses to increased IAP in a porcine model. At 25 mmHg IAP, cardiac index, and urine output were significantly decreased and PRA and aldosterone significantly increased compared to baseline. The animals were then volume loaded until the cardiac index was returned to baseline values. Intravascular volume expansion significantly increased urine output above baseline even though IAP was maintained at 25 mmHg. PRA and aldosterone levels fell with volume expansion, but remained above baseline levels. Subsequent abdominal decompression fur-

ther decreased both PRA and aldosterone levels. There were no significant changes in ANF at any time point. Renal venous pressures were significantly elevated with the increased IAP.

These investigators postulated a central role for increased PRA and aldosterone in the renal dysfunction associated with acutely elevated IAP. Furthermore, they suggested that the elevation of renal venous pressure secondary to the elevated IAP may be causally related to the significant increases in PRA and aldosterone levels observed. The findings of significant increases in both PRA and aldosterone with acute increases in IAP are consistent with, and supported by, the findings of previous investigators. Shenasky and Gillenwater [14] reported that urinary sodium and chloride concentrations decreased significantly with increased IAP and returned to normal with abdominal decompression. The role of sodium excretion was more severely reduced in their study than could be accounted for by the diminished delivery of sodium to the renal tubules. Also, urinary potassium levels increased with rising IAP. These urinary ion concentration changes are consistent with the increased aldosterone levels with elevated IAP demonstrated in the Bloomfield study.

The adverse effects of increased IAP on renal function have also been demonstrated experimentally in normal human subjects. Bradley et al. [15] demonstrated marked decreases in RBF, GFR, and tubular reabsorption of glucose by abdominal compression to a pressure of 20 mmHg in the inferior vena cava. Renal venous pressure increased from 5.8 mmHg to 18.3 mmHg, while mean arterial pressure was not altered by the elevated IAP. GFR decreased to the same extent as the fall in effective renal plasma flow, indicating that the filtration fraction was unchanged.

Clinical Studies

The clinical studies on the hemodynamic effects of acute increases in IAP have largely focused on post-surgical or trauma patients. These clinical reports are limited by a number of factors:
a) in many patients, increased IAP was due to continued bleeding in the abdominal cavity or retroperitoneum and thus had an additive effect on renal hemodynamics;
b) renal function assessment was limited to either urine output or to changes in serum creatinine; and
c) the baseline renal function in these patients was not known, but was presumably normal.

In one of the earlier clinical reports, Richards et al. [16] reported an anuric renal failure in four patients in association with increased IAP from postoperative hemorrhage. The mean hemodynamic parameters in these patients included a cardiac index of 3.68 l/min per square meter, a pulmonary wedge pressure of 18.7 mmHg, and a mean arterial pressure of 110 mmHg. The decreased urine output was refractory to fluid boluses and diuretics. However, polyuria and resolution of the renal failure occurred in each patient in response to operative decompression of the abdomen. Interestingly, bilateral ureteral catheters were placed in one patient with no resolution of the anuria. In another patient a renal arterial isotope study demonstrated normal bilateral renal artery perfusion. Apparently IAP was not measured in the clinical study by Richards et al.

Cullen et al. [17] reported on the cardiovascular and renal effects of increased intra-abdominal pressure in six patients. The mean IAP was 51 ± 7 cm H_2O (SE). Cardiac output was 4.7 ± 1 l/min prevolume challenge and 5.6 ± 1.2 l/min postvolume challenge. Wedge pressures were 25 ± 4 and 28 ± 4 pre- and postvolume challenge. In contrast, left ventricular end-diastolic volume was somewhat small (64 ± 14 ml). Oliguria (urine output < 10 ml/h) was present and did not respond to the fluid challenge. However, surgical decompression of the abdomen improved urine output within 15 min. Additionally, several other reports corroborate the findings noted in these clinical studies [18, 19].

Finally, Sugrue [20] demonstrated the clinical significance of the association between raised IAP and renal impairment in patients admitted to the intensive care unit following laparotomy. In their prospective study, Sugrue et al. noted increased IAP (bladder pressure > 20 mmHg) in 33%. Renal impairment (defined as a serum creatinine > 1.3 mg/l or an increase in serum creatinine > 1 mg/l within 72 h of surgery) was observed in 33%. Of note, 20 of 24, or 69%, of patients who developed impaired renal function had raised IAP.

Although increased IAP may negatively impact renal blood by decreasing cardiac output, it also has direct adverse effects on renal hemodynamics and function. The prior experimental studies and clinical reports document impaired renal function with raised IAP, especially with IAP greater than 20–25 mmHg. Of note, the report by Chiu et al. previously cited suggests adverse effects on the renal circulation with intra-abdominal pressures currently employed for laparoscopic procedures. As usual practice all patients should have urine output monitored intraoperatively during laparoscopic procedures. Patients with compromised cardiac or renal function may benefit from monitoring and optimization of cardiac output during advanced laparoscopic procedures. Pharmacologic blockade of the hormonal response to increased IAP may help modulate the associated adverse hemodynamic consequences. This may be especially useful in the compromised patient undergoing a potentially long laparoscopic procedure.

Summary

In summary, the following points should be noted (Table 1):
- Acute increases in IAP negatively impact RBF due to changes in cardiac output and renal vascular resistance noted with elevated IAP.
- Correcting cardiac output to normal or supranormal values when IAP is > 20 mmHg does not restore renal function to normal. The effectiveness of maintaining cardiac output at normal or higher levels of renal function when IAP < 15 mmHg is uncertain.
- Increases in renal vascular resistance account for the direct effects of increased IAP on RBF and function.

Table 1. Renal physiologic mani-
festations of increased intra-abdominal pressure (IAP)

Experimental studies
    Oliguria/anuria
    ↓ Renal blood flow
    ↓ GFR
    Increased renal vascular resistance
    ↓ Urinary sodium
    ↑ Urine/plasma osmolarity

Clinical reports
    Oliguria/anuria
    ↑ Serum creatinine
    ↓ Creatinine clearance

GFR, glomerular filtration rate.

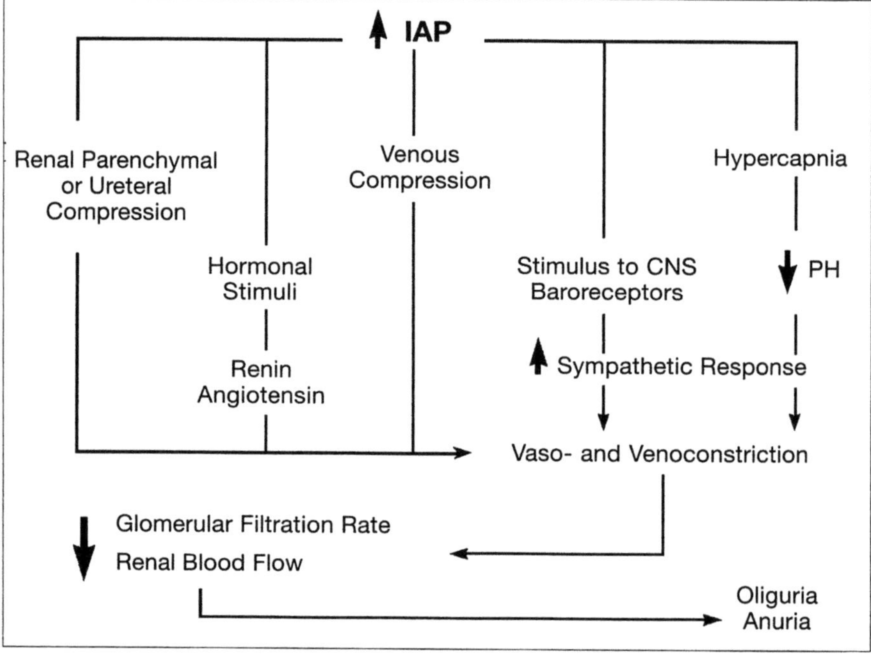

Fig. 1. Summary of effects of increase in intra-abdominal pressure (IAP)

- Renal venous pressure changes coincide with increases in IAP. Renal venous
  hypertension increases renal vascular resistance by obstructing renal venous
  outflow.
- Increases in renal vascular resistance with IAP may in part be due to neural,
  hormonal, or intrinsic influences (Fig. 1).

References

1. Thorington JM, Schmidt CF (1923) A study of urinary output and blood pressure changes resulting in experimental ascites. Am J Med Sci 165:880–886
2. Dunn MJ, Hood VL (1977) Prostaglandins and the kidney. Am J Physiol 233:169–184
3. Garrison RN, Wilson MA, Matheson PJ, Spain DA (1995) Nitric oxide mediates redistribution of intrarenal blood flow during bacteremia. J Trauma 39:90–97
4. Caldwell CB, Ricotta JJ (1987) Changes in visceral blood flow with elevated intraabdominal pressure. J Surg Res 43:14–20
5. Barnes GE, Laine GA, Giam PY et al (1985) Cardiovascular responses to elevation of intraabdominal hydratic pressure. Am J Physiol 248:R208–R213
6. Harman PK, Kron IL, McLachlon HD et al (1982) Elevated intraabdominal pressure and renal function. Ann Surg 196:594–597
7. Chiu AW, Chang LS, Birkett DH, Babayan RK (1996) A porcine model for renal hemodynamic study during laparoscopy. J Surg Res 60:61–68
8. Vaughan ED, Shenasky JH, Gillenwater JY (1971) Mechanisms of acute hemodynamic response to ureteral occlusion. Invest Urol 9:109–18
9. Stone HH, Fulenwider JT (1977) Renal decapsulation in the prevention of post-ischemic oliguria. Ann Surg 186:343–355
10. Bloomfield GL, Blocher CR, Fakhry IF et al (1996) Elevated intra-abdominal pressure upregulates the renin–angiotensin–aldosterone system. J Trauma 41:193 (abstr)
11. Julius S, Sanchez R, Malayan S et al (1982) Sustained blood pressure elevation to lower body compression in pigs and dogs. Hypertension 4:782–788
12. Price HL (1960) Effects of carbon dioxide on the cardiovascular system. Anesthesiology 21:652–657
13. Le Roith D, Bark H, Nyska M, Glick SN (1982) The effects of abdominal pressure in plasma antidiuretic hormone levels in the dog. J Surg Res 32:65–69
14. Shenasky JH, Gillinwater JY (1972) The renal hemodynamic and functional effects of external counter pressure. Surg Gynecol Obset 134:253–258
15. Bradley SE, Bradley GP (1947) The effects of increased intraabdominal pressures on renal function in man. J Clin Invest 26:1010–22
16. Richards WO, Scovill W, Shin B, Reed W (1983) Acute renal failure associated with increased intraabdominal pressure. Ann Surg 197:183–187
17. Cullen DJ, Coyle JP, Teplick R, Lang MC (1989) Cardiovascular, pulmonary, and renal effects of massively increased intra-abdominal pressure in critically ill patients. Crit Care Med 17:118–121
18. Platell C, Hall J, Dobb G (1990) Impaired renal function due to raised intraabdominal pressure. Intensive Care Med 16:328–329
19. Smith JH, Merrell RC, Raffin TA (1985) Reversal of post-operative anuria by decompressive celiotomy. Arch Intern Med 145:553–554
20. Sugrue M, Buist MD, Houriham F et al (1995) Prospective study of intraabdominal hypertension and renal function after laparotomy. Br J Surg 82:235–238

8 Respiratory Changes During Carbon Dioxide Pneumoperitoneum

S. Steigerwald, H. Bockhorn, and R. Denhardt

Introduction

In contrast to conventional surgery laparoscopic procedures are considered to be minimally invasive. Initially, laparoscopies were of brief duration and were usually performed on otherwise healthy gynecologic patients [1, 2]. Since the improvement of laparoscopic techniques more extended procedures have been performed. The patient population undergoing laparoscopic intervention has also significantly changed. The amount of high-risk patients with cardiopulmonary impairments has increased. When performing laparoscopic surgery, a carbon dioxide pneumoperitoneum is usually established. Experiments have shown that carbon dioxide insufflation into the peritoneal cavity and the subsequent increase in intra-abdominal pressure results in significant respiratory changes due to hypercapnia and diminished alveolar ventilation in the lower lung lobes. Pathophysiological aspects of increased carbon dioxide absorption, as well as aspects of respiratory changes, especially in patients suffering from chronic pulmonary diseases, and the role of positive end-expiratory pressure application will be elucidated.

Hypercapnia

The peritoneum is a serous membrane composed of a monocellular layer of flattened mesothelial cells resting on a thin layer of fibroelastic tissue. The diaphragmatic mesothelium possesses intercellular openings, called stomata, which are the primary route of absorption of particulate material from the peritoneal cavity [3]. The vasculature of the peritoneum is scanty. In a study of its microvascular anatomy, human visceral peritoneum was shown to derive its blood supply from arterioles that are passed to it from underlying bowel muscle vessels. These arterioles supply a capillary plexus containing two layers of closely packed long, straight vessels that are oriented at right angles to each other [4] (Fig. 1, nos. 3–6). The total peritoneal surface area is nearly 2 m², but the functional absorptive surface area is thought to be only about 1 m².

The peritoneum transports water, electrolytes, small molecules such as gases, and certain macromolecules. Though controversy exists regarding precise mechanisms and pathways, our knowledge of peritoneal membrane transport functions has recently increased, based on studies conducted in patients undergoing intermittent and chronic peritoneal dialysis. The movement of fluid across the

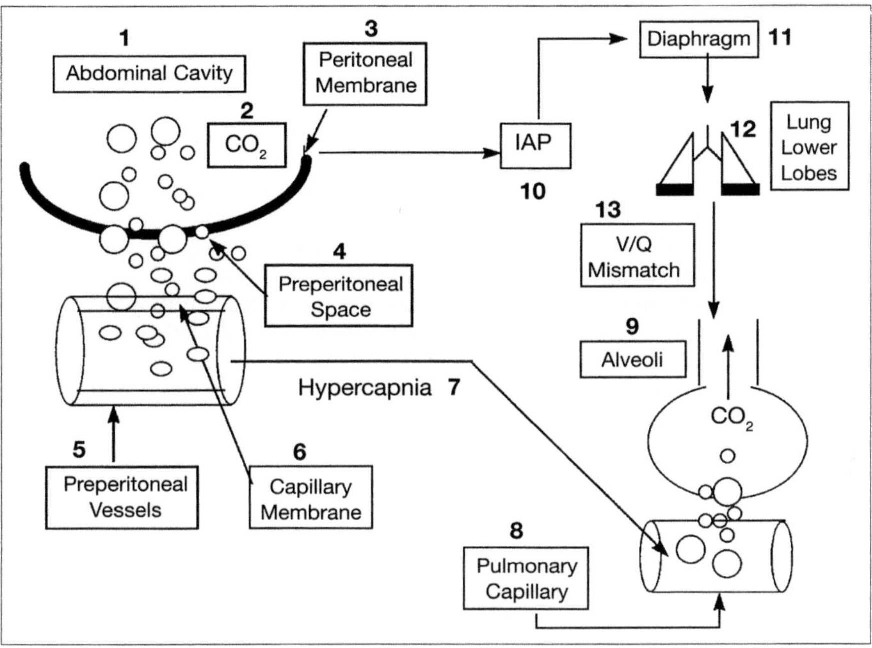

Fig. 1. The peritoneal cavity (*1*) is able to absorb gaseous molecules (*2*) by diffusion. Through the peritoneal membrane (*3*), preperitoneal space (*4*) and capillary membrane (*6*), carbon dioxide molecules can enter the peritoneal vessels (*5*), causing hypercapnia (*7*) by increasing the carbon dioxide blood tension. As a compensation, excretion of carbon dioxide through the alveoli will be increased (*8,9*). When applying carbon dioxide pneumoperitoneum, intra-abdominal pressure (IAP, *10*) will increase simultaneously, causing diminished excursion of the diaphragm (*11*) and compression of the lower lung lobes (*12*), resulting in decreased tidal volume and a ventilation–perfusion mismatch (*13*) with increased shunt and dead space volume

peritoneal membrane is bidirectional between the peritoneal cavity and plasma. Transport of small molecules across the membrane takes place by convection and diffusion [5].

Convection has been demonstrated to occur with small solutes such as urea and creatinine, while diffusion is more pronounced for small molecules such as potassium and sodium. Electrolytes, proteins, and many other endogenous and exogenous materials are freely absorbed. Absorption appears not to be affected by blood flow to the peritoneal membrane. Factors that are thought to influence absorption are intra-abdominal pressure, temperature, dehydration, and increased portal pressure. Experimental work has shown that the stomata open and close with relaxation and contraction of the diaphragm, suggesting that patency may be altered by the respiratory cycle [5]. The stomata remain open in the presence of increased intra-abdominal pressure, this being an adaptive mechanism to facilitate removal of fluids and gases from the peritoneal cavity [5, 6] (Fig. 1, no. 10).

During laparoscopic surgery a pneumoperitoneum commonly established by 100% carbon dioxide insufflation into the peritoneal cavity is necessary (Fig. 1, nos. 1–2). Numerous experimental studies have been done to elucidate the effect of carbon dioxide pneumoperitoneum on human physiology, especially on respiratory changes. Most of the early experimental data was obtained on healthy females undergoing laparoscopy for gynecologic disease [1, 2]. In this group the intraperitoneal insufflation of carbon dioxide resulted in a significant rise in arterial carbon dioxide tension and a significant decrease in arterial pH [2, 7]. This was explained by the fact that the peritoneal space is a closed, collapsible body cavity that normally contains little serous fluid.

After introduction of carbon dioxide into the peritoneal cavity two immediate effects could be observed. Firstly, the pressure within the cavity was raised to a level that depends on the gas introduced and on the compliance of the cavity (Fig. 1, no. 10). Secondly, gaseous interchange started to take place between the gas and the peritoneal vessels (Fig. 1, nos. 5–6). During this period the carbon dioxide in the cavity came to an equilibrium with the blood gases. Therefore, insufflation of 100% carbon dioxide in the peritoneal cavity produced a partial pressure difference between the peritoneal vessels and the peritoneal cavity of 670 mmHg at atmospheric pressure. Differences in carbon dioxide partial pressures between the capillary blood and the peritoneal cavity are one of the major driving forces for diffusion from the peritoneal cavity into the blood stream during carbon dioxide pneumoperitoneum [8]. Other important factors are the amount of surface available for diffusion, as well as the thickness of cell layers that has to be passed by the gas molecules (Fick's first law of diffusion) [9]. Therefore, this high partial pressure difference caused a rapid flow of carbon dioxide gas entering the circulation. An increase in arterial carbon dioxide tension has been measured (Fig. 1, no. 7). The alveolar membrane is about 25 times more patent for carbon dioxide than for oxygen. Therefore, most of the carbon dioxide will be carried by circulation to the lung where it is excreted (Fig. 1, nos. 8–9). Subsequently the plasma carbon dioxide concentration decreases and the gas molecules have been replaced by carbon dioxide emerging from erythrocytes. These intracellular molecules are produced from bicarbonate ions by enzymatic reactions. All these previously described reactions are very rapid and efficient in healthy individuals, leading to higher tidal volumes and breathing frequencies. During anesthesia, therefore, controlled ventilation to maintain adequate oxygen values is essential [9].

That the increase of frequency and tidal volume is an effect of increasing hypercapnia and subsequent respiratory acidosis and not a result of insufficient ventilation during surgery has been proved in many experiments [1, 2, 8]. Preventing respiratory compensation by not adjusting minute ventilation showed increasing hypercapnia.

The absence of any significant change in the level of bicarbonates or base excess during these experiments confirms that hypercapnia and acidosis were entirely respiratory and not of metabolic cause [8]. Using other gases for pneumoperitoneum such as helium, or using mechanical retractors instead of gas insufflation indicated that hypercapnia and acidosis can probably be avoided during laparoscopic surgery [10].

Because carbon dioxide is capable of penetrating all cell membranes and ultimately increasing intracellular hydrogen ion concentration (respiratory-caused intracellular acidosis) by changing the carbon dioxide-bicarbonate-hydrogen ion equilibrium, it can exert systemic toxic effects if its excretion is impaired. Enzymatic transformation of the gas into bicarbonate in stomach and bones as well as activation of multiple buffer systems in blood and kidney cells in order to avoid dangerously elevated hydrogen ion concentration, can be accelerated but cannot substitute pulmonary elimination [8, 11, 12].

Ventilation-Perfusion Mismatch

The main process which takes place in the alveoli is blood arterialization. Herein the oxygen partial pressure of the capillary alveolar blood increases, while the carbon dioxide partial pressure decreases. Factors which influence this are alveolar ventilation, blood perfusion of the lung, and finally ventilation distribution. In healthy subjects not all parts of the lung are equally ventilated. Normally, in the vertical position the upper parts of the lung are less ventilated than the lower lobes. This leads to a decrease in arterialization and an increase in carbon dioxide partial pressure in the arterial blood. As a reflex alveolar capillaries of less ventilated alveoli are constricted and the arteriovenous shunt volume minimized. At the same time dead space volume will be reduced [13]. Insufflation of the peritoneal cavity causes distention and increases in intra-abdominal pressure, which can have a significant effect on mechanically supported ventilation. It decreases diaphragmatic excursion and increases the pressure forced on the lower lung lobes, resulting in decreased end-expiratory tidal volume (Fig. 1, nos. 11–12). At the same time, the number of less ventilated alveoli increases, resulting in an increased ventilation-perfusion mismatch, causing elevated dead space and shunt volume [13] (Fig. 1, no. 13).

Lung Diseases

Emphysema, a disease representing one characteristic expression of advanced chronic obstructive pulmonary disease, is characterized by enlarged air spaces produced by a complex process of elastic tissue destruction, alveolar wall breakdown, and coalescence of damaged alveoli, resulting in impaired alveolar ventilation and gas exchange [6]. Expiration is impaired by collapsing airway ductuli, concluding in hypoventilation. At the same time, the alveolar capillaries are compressed, resulting in increased dead space [8].

In restrictive pulmonary disease, on the other hand, alveoli are replaced by fibrotic tissue, decreasing the surface available for diffusion (decreased diffusion capacity). Gas exchange is also impaired by lost lung compliance. Increased arteriovenous shunt volumes are due to lost contact between alveoli and capillary blood vessels [11, 12].

Few experiments have been carried out to elucidate the influence of carbon dioxide pneumoperitoneum on patients suffering from chronic lung disease. In a canine model chronic obstructive lung disease was established by pepain inhalation treatment, causing progressive panlobular emphysema. The dogs underwent laparoscopic surgery using carbon dioxide pneumoperitoneum. It could been demonstrated that subjects suffering from chronic obstructive pulmonary disease exposed to 15-mmHg pneumoperitoneum retained carbon dioxide disproportionately to normal subjects due to impaired carbon dioxide excretion abilities [14].

Positive End-Expiratory Pressure

The lung is separated from the thoracic cavity by the pleural space. The pressure in the pleural space is negative during normal breathing. Transpulmonary pressure, distending pressure across the lung, and lung compliance determine lung volume; positive end-expiratory pressure (PEEP) causes an increase in lung volume at end expiration, i.e., an increase in functional residual capacity. The decrease in functional residual capacity is the most physiologically significant aspect of pulmonary diseases, manifesting, for example, as alveolar collapse in chronic obstructive diseases [15]. If blood flow continues past the collapsed alveoli, that portion of the total pulmonary blood flow never passes oxygen-containing alveoli and consequently remains desaturated. When the desaturated blood joins the remainder of the pulmonary blood flow, the resultant systemic partial oxygen pressure is lower. The blood which flows through the lung without being oxygenated is referred to as intrapulmonary shunt volume. PEEP can increase the end-expiratory lung volume, improving, subsequently, the ventilation of poorly ventilated or collapsed alveoli, decreasing intrapulmonary shunt volumes, and finally increasing systemic partial oxygen pressure. Lung compliance, as pathologically changed in restrictive pulmonary disease, is a measure of the elasticity of the lung, defined as "change in volume divided by change in distending pressure." When PEEP is applied previously, collapsed alveoli can be inflated and compliance may be improved. Nevertheless, compliance can also be decreased during PEEP ventilation as a result of overdistension of alveoli, alveolar rupture, and surfactant inactivation. For this reason, the effects of PEEP on lung compliance are a point of controversy [16].

PEEP can have important effects on the distribution of ventilation and perfusion in the lung. Ventilation-perfusion mismatch frequently occurs in pulmonary diseases [16]. Ventilation in excess of perfusion is manifest as increase in dead space; perfusion in excess of ventilation is manifest as increased shunt volume and decreased partial oxygen pressure [15]. Measurements of the effects of PEEP on dead space are conflicting: increased, as well as decreased, dead space volume by applying PEEP ventilation has been found by several investigators [12]. Establishing carbon dioxide pneumoperitoneum during laparoscopic surgery results in multiple respiratory changes. Hypercapnia, respiratory acidosis, higher tidal volumes, and increasing frequency have previously been described [16]. As laparoscopic techniques have become more sophisticated extended laparoscopic surgery has been performed on high-risk patients with reduced cardiopulmonary reserves. Usually, PEEP has been added to conventional mechanical ventilation in patients prone to develop postoperative pulmonary complications. In particular, patients with diminished functional residual capacity might theoretically benefit from PEEP during the period in which increased intra-abdominal pressure compresses the basal lung areas. An increase in intra-abdominal pressure decreases diaphragmatic excursion, resulting in decreased end-expiratory tidal volume, which may in turn increase carbon dioxide retention [14]. Experiments on canine models indicate that the application of PEEP and carbon dioxide pneumoperitoneum simultaneously significantly increases the fractional end-tidal carbon dioxide and the arterial carbon dioxide tension due to intra-abdominal resorption of the gas [14]. Application of carbon dioxide pneumoperitoneum alone results in a lesser increase in end-tidal carbon dioxide. Explanations of these results are difficult to obtain. Investigators have found increased dead space volume in dogs with normal lungs [14]. In animals with abnormal lungs measurements of dead space volumes are contradictory. If conducting airways are increased in size, if normal alveoli are overextended, or if perfusion to normal alveoli is decreased due to alveolar distention, an overall increase in dead space volume has been measured. If a constant tidal volume is better distributed with respect to perfusion as a result of the relief of atelectasis, a decrease in dead space volume has been measured by application of PEEP. Applying PEEP to the normal lung may cause overdistension of alveoli and an increase in pulmonary vascular resistance, diverting blood flow to the less ventilated lung areas and resulting in increased intrapulmonary shunt volume and decreased arterial oxygen tension. Furthermore, on the application of PEEP increased blood flow to diseased lung lobes has been observed and subsequently increased shunt volume has been measured.

Conclusions

Carbon dioxide pneumoperitoneum during laparoscopic surgery has significant effects on the patient's ventilation. Due to gas absorption through the peritoneal cavity membrane the arterial carbon dioxide tension significantly increases, leading to respiratory acidosis. Tidal volume, end-tidal carbon dioxide pressure, and breathing frequency have to be increased as an effect of hypercapnia [17]. At the same time, increasing pressure forced on the lower lung lobes during pneumoperitoneum decreases the number of sufficiently ventilated alveoli, resulting in an increase in ventilation-perfusion mismatch with elevated dead space and shunt volume. Mechanical ventilation has to be adjusted in order to compensate for these effects and to ensure sufficient oxygen supply during laparoscopic surgery. The application of PEEP ventilation seems to be beneficial.

Special problems occur as laparoscopic techniques become more sophisticated and extended laparoscopic procedures are carried out on patients with cardiopulmonary impairments. Chronic obstructive and restrictive diseases lead to inefficient carbon dioxide excretion. Particularly in this group of subjects the benefit of PEEP during artificial ventilation is a point of controversy.

Taking all aspects into consideration, laparoscopic surgery using carbon dioxide pneumoperitoneum has to be done as fast as possible in order to keep gas resorption time and pulmonary stress as short as possible. At the end of surgery carbon dioxide should be removed as completely as possible in order to avoid additional carbon dioxide absorption after surgery. Since the human body has a tremendous carbon dioxide storage capacity (120 l) [18], a hypercapnic hangover has to be taken into consideration, thus necessitating close cardiopulmonary monitoring of the patient.

References

1. Lewis DG, Ryder W, Burn K, Wheldon TJ, Tacchi D (1972) Laparscopy: an investigation during spontaneous ventilation with halothane. Br J Anaesth 44:685–690
2. Motew M, Ivankovich AD, Bieniarz J, Albrecht RF, Zahed B, Scommegna A, Silverman B (1973) Cardiovascular effects and acid-base and blood gas changes during laparoscopy. Am J Obstet Gynecol (7):1002–1012
3. Tsilibary EC, Wissig SL (1983) Lymphatic absorption from the peritoneal cavity: regulation of patency of medothelial stomata. Microvasc Res 25:22–39
4. Northaver JMA, Williams EDF (1980) The investigation of small vessel anatomy by scanning electron microscopy of resin casts. A description of the technique and examples of its use in the study of the microvasculature of the peritoneum and bile duct wall. J Anat 130:43–54
5. Flessner MF, Dedrick RL (1984) A distributed model of peritoneal-plasma transport: theoretical considerations. Am J Physiol 246:R597–R607
6. Schwartz SJ, Shires GT, Spencer FC (1989) Principles of surgery, 5th edn, vol 2. MacGraw Hill, New York, pp 1459–1489
7. Alexander GD, Brown EM (1969) Physiologic alterations during pelvic laparoscopy. Am J Obstet Gynecol 105:1078–1081
8. El-Minawi MF, Wahbi MCO, El-Bagouri IS, Sharawi M, El-Mallah SY (1981) Physiologic changes during CO_2 and N_2O pneumoperitoneum in diagnostic lapararoscopy. J Reprod Med 26:338–346
9. Schmidt RF, Thaws G (1983) Physiologie des Menschen. Springer, Berlin Heidelberg New York, pp 522–526
10. McDermott JP, Regan MC, Page R, Stokes MA, Barry K, Moriarty DC, Cavshay PE, Fitzpatrick JM, Gorey TF (1993) Cardiorespiratory effects of laparoscopy with and without gas insufflation. Arch Surg 130:984–988
11. Lang F (1983) Pathophysiologie und Pathobiochemie. Ferdinand Encke, Stuttgart, pp 61–90
12. Luz CM, Polarz H, Böhrer H, Hundt G, Dörsam J, Martin E (1994) Hemodynamic and respiratory effects of pneumoperitoneun and PEEP during laparoscopic pelvic lymphadenectomy in dogs. Surg Endosc 8:25–27
13. Wittgen CM, Andrus CH, Fitzgerald SD, Baudendistel LJ, Dahms TE, Kaminski DL (1991) Analysis of the hemodynamic and ventilatory effects of laparoscopic cholecystectomy. Arch Surg 126:997–1001
14. Fitzgerald SD, Andrus CH, Baudendistel LJ, Dahms TE, Kaminski DL (1992) Hypercarbia during carbon dioxide pneumoperitoneum. Am J Surg 163:186–190
15. Tyler DC (1983) Positive end-expiratory pressure: a review. Crit Care Med 11:300–305
16. Burchard KW, Clombor DM, McLeod MK, Slothman GJ, Gann DS (1985) Positive end-expiratory pressure with increased intra-abdominal pressure. Surg Gynecol Obstet 161:313–318
17. McMahon AJ, Baxter JN, Kenny G, O'Dwyer PJ (1993) Ventilatory and blood gas changes during laparoscopic and open cholecystectomy. Br J Surg 80:1252–1254
18. Ho HS, Gunther RA, Wolfe BM (1992) Intraperitoneal carbon dioxide insufflation and cardiopulmonary functions. Arch Surg 127:928–933

9 Cardiovascular Changes During Laparoscopy

B.A. Laureano, C.H. Andrus, and D.L. Kaminski

Introduction

Initially, a brief gynecologic diagnostic tool in young, healthy patients, longer and more complex laparoscopic surgery has gained increasing popularity in recent years. In the late 1980s, laparoscopy was reintroduced to the general surgeon with laparoscopic cholecystectomy. Since then the use of laparoscopy has grown to include many intra-abdominal procedures. As the benefits of laparoscopic surgery, predominantly laparoscopic cholecystectomy, became apparent, so did the application. The patient population undergoing laparoscopic surgery has been extended to an older group of patients, with more underlying illnesses and an overall higher surgical risk; an increasing number of procedures of variable complexity and requiring substantially longer procedural times are being carried out. With more high-risk patients and longer operating times, the potential morbidity of laparoscopic surgery has become increasingly significant.

To provide an adequate visualization of the surgical field, the anterior abdominal wall is elevated in the majority of laparoscopies by creating an artificial positive-pressure pneumoperitoneum. This chapter will focus on the hemodynamic changes associated with increased intra-abdominal pressure with gas insufflation of the abdomen and discuss the effects of the various gases themselves.

Carbon Dioxide Insufflation

Currently, CO_2 is the most commonly employed pneumoperitoneum agent because it is nonflammable, readily available, and highly diffusible. There are two distinct methods of influence on the hemodynamic system:

1. Systemic effects of the insufflation gas and
2. mechanical effects of increased intra-abdominal pressure. Initially, it was thought that there were negligible systemic effects from intra-abdominal insufflation of CO_2.

However, it was soon realized that the absence of noticeable effects was due to well-functioning physiologic compensatory mechanisms. Carbon dioxide gas is systemically absorbed from the peritoneal surface resulting in hypercapnia [1, 20]. Systemically dissolved CO_2 results in serum acidosis correctable by hyperventilation. Increased procedure time with resultant increased CO_2 absorption and an individual's diminished respiratory capacity for CO_2 elimination due to underlying pulmonary disease, can overcome the compensatory mechanisms resulting in detectable hypercapnia and serum acidosis [30].

Hypercapnia

Hypercapnia and the resultant acidosis have numerous systemic effects. Possibly by lowering an individual's arrhythmia threshold, hypercapnia has been shown to increase the incidence of cardiac arrhythmias [26]. Mild hypercapnia can cause sympathetic stimulation that leads to an increase in heart rate and peripheral vasoconstriction, resulting in increased blood pressure and increased cardiac output [17, 24]. Severe hypercapnia can exert a negative inotropic effect on the heart, resulting in a depression of left ventricular function [28].

There have been several studies attempting to separate the pneumoperitoneum effects of hypercapnia from increased intra-abdominal pressure. In a chronic obstructive pulmonary disease (COPD) canine model, increased arterial pressure, increased pulmonary artery pressure, and a resultant increase in cardiac output was noted with pneumoperitoneal insufflation [6]. It was concluded that the hemodynamic changes were due to increased abdominal pressure as the changes were similar with both CO_2 and helium insufflation. However, in a pig model where CO_2 insufflation was also compared to helium insufflation, the CO_2 pneumoperitoneum produced an elevated systemic blood pressure, a slight increase in heart rate, and a decrease in cardiac output when compared to the effects of the helium pneumoperitoneum [13]. These changes were attributed to CO_2 absorption from the peritoneal surface, as they were not seen in the helium insufflation.

A more recent study in a pig model specifically looked at hypercapnia versus increased intra-abdominal pressure, comparing CO_2 with nitrogen insufflation [8]. The hemodynamic changes observed were a decrease in stroke volume with a compensatory tachycardia that maintained the cardiac index at approximately baseline levels. In the CO_2 insufflation group, hypercapnia and acidemia quickly developed, along with increased pulmonary CO_2 excretion and oxygen consumption. The authors concluded that the observed hemodynamic effects were due almost entirely to CO_2 absorption, as no changes were observed in the nitrogen group. Interestingly, an observation was noted regarding the persistence of certain changes following desufflation of the abdomen. Stroke volume was depressed for up to 40 min into the recovery period, possibly reflecting the temporally delayed redistribution of interstitial CO_2 gas into the serum with subsequent respiratory excretion. This persistent low stroke volume, in combination with resolution of the tachycardia, led to a decrease in cardiac index during the recovery period. None of these changes were noticed with the nitrogen insufflation. CO_2 insufflation has been studied in other reports, but not in comparison to increased intra-abdominal pressure by another method. There are many examples of studies in which hemodynamic changes are seen in CO_2 insufflation; however, they cannot be attributed to either CO_2 absorption or intra-abdominal pressure independently as there were no appropriate comparisons performed (Table 1).

The information obtained from animal studies would suggest that in normal patients the hemodynamic effects of laparoscopy with CO_2 insufflation are primarily due to CO_2 absorption and the resultant serum acid-base changes. In patients with chronic illnesses such as COPD, the hemodynamic changes are accentuated with increased intra-abdominal pressure being more relevant.

In patients with known limited compensatory mechanisms, as in concomitant cardiac or pulmonary disease, the side effects of hypercapnia and increased intra-abdominal pressure can be significant [25, 30]. In this patient population, invasive cardiopulmonary monitoring may be warranted during laparoscopy.

Mechanical Effects of Increased Intra-abdominal Pressure

During laparoscopic surgery, abdominal wall retraction and peritoneal expansion are needed to visualize the surgical field; this is usually produced by gaseous distension methods associated with increased intra-abdominal pressure. Increased abdominal pressure has several effects, most notably decreased venous return secondary to the compression of venous structures. The positioning of patients during laparoscopic procedures can also affect venous return: in a "head-down" or Trendelenburg position, a positive effect on venous return may be seen; while in a "head-up" or reverse-Trendelenburg position, a negative effect on venous return may be observed. Intravascular volume status has some relationship to the effect of the intraperitoneal pressure on central filling pressures. High intra-abdominal pressures augment venous return in subjects with high right-sided pressures maintaining a patent inferior vena cava (IVC), whereas low right-sided pressures lead to a compressed IVC and a decrease in venous return [10, 25].

Metabolic Effects of Increased Intra-abdominal Pressure

Hypercapnia is known to have a stimulatory effect on hemodynamics. When the intra-abdominal pressure is raised (40 mmHg), however, the decrease in venous return overcomes the stimulant effect and there is a decrease in cardiac output [21]. An increase in systemic vascular resistance observed in canine experiments is possibly explained by compression of the abdominal aorta, increased sympathetic activity with arteriolar constriction, or increased splanchnic venous resistance [11]. Intravascular volume status has some relationship to the effect of the intraperitoneal pressure on central filling pressures.

Effects of Increased Intra-abdominal Pressure on Cardiac Output

In the majority of studies, the overall hemodynamic changes produced by laparoscopy show similar trends with increased central filling pressures, increased arterial pressures, and increased systemic vascular resistance. The effect on cardiac output differs in these studies possibly due to the different methods of its measurement [16, 27], different volume status of the subject [13], or different responses of vascular beds to the effects of vasoconstrictors (i.e., dog vs pig vs human). These studies show increased [7, 18], or decreased [19, 21, 25, 29] cardiac output (Table 1).

Table 1. Collective results of the effects of CO_2 pneumoperitoneum on hemodynamic variables

Reference	Subject	SVR	SV	HR	CO	CVP	BP
[18]	Pig	N/A	↑	↑	↑	—	N/A
[19]	Human	N/A	N/A	—	↓	↑	↑
[5]	Pig	—	↓	↑	—	N/A	N/A
[21]	Human	↑	—	↑	↓	↑	↑
[29]	Dog	↑	↓	N/A	↓	—	—
[17]	Human	N/A	N/A	↑	—	↑	↑
[25]	Human	↓	N/A	↓	↓	N/A	↑

N/A indicates that the parameter was not measured; ↑ indicates an icrease; ↓ indicates a decrease; — indicates that there was no change.
SVR, systemic vascular resistance; SV, stroke volume; HR, heart rate; CO, cardiac output; CVP, central venous pressure; BP, blood pressure.

Effects of Increased Intra-abdominal Pressure on Organ Perfusion

Preliminary studies of increased intra-abdominal pressure have demonstrated a negative effect on abdominal organ perfusion. In a canine study comparing CO_2 versus helium insufflation, effects of intra-abdominal pressure resulting in visceral ischemia were observed unrelated to the insufflating gas [11]. Little effect on renal blood flow has been noted with CO_2 pneumoperitoneum [11,12]. The effect of intra-abdominal pressure on organ perfusion requires further investigation.

Effects of Increased Intra-abdominal Pressure in High-Risk Cardiac Disease

The clinical evaluation of patients with high-risk cardiac disease (American Society of Anesthesiologists' categories III or IV) undergoing laparoscopy produced several important conclusions. The preoperative risk classification was not predictive of the hemodynamic compromise. Complex hemodynamic changes take place with the induction of anesthesia followed by abrupt elevation in intra-abdominal pressure, resulting in patients with fixed coronary lesions being at risk of coronary ischemia. Volume loading with intravenous fluids prior to anesthetic induction seems to offset the effects of increased intra-abdominal pressure considering the increased venous return in a state with high right-sided pressures. Volume loading must be done in moderation, however, as too much volume in some patients may lead to a decline in cardiac function. Finally, the most sensitive measure of the hemodynamic and cardiovascular status is the mixed venous oxygen saturations [25]. There are many potential variables ultimately affecting hemodynamics that as yet have not been completely evaluated in order to fully define the causes of hemodynamic changes associated with laparoscopy.

Alternative Gases or Methods

Several gases have been proposed or utilized for insufflation of the abdomen: carbon dioxide, nitrous oxide, air, oxygen, argon, and helium. Some of these gases (oxygen, nitrous oxide, air) can support combustion precluding the employment of electrocautery. CO_2 is most commonly used at present because it does not support combustion in the presence of electrocautery, it is inexpensive, and is highly soluble with minimal risk of embolism. Nitrous oxide continues to be employed in diagnostic laparoscopies and in those cases not requiring cautery. It is non-irritating to the peritoneum, unlike CO_2, and thus can be utilized with local anesthetic techniques. As previously discussed, CO_2 does have physiologic effects, including acid-base and hormonal changes, and for this reason an alternative insufflating gas is continuously being sought. At present, the most promising alternative gas for abdominal insufflation is helium.

Helium

Helium is a readily available, nonflammable, physiologically-inert gas. It has been studied in several animal models and patients. In the animal models the effects observed during helium pneumoperitoneum were attributed to the increased intra-abdominal pressure, including decreased venous return and increased ventilation pressures [11]. With helium insufflation, there were no changes in the partial pressure of carbon dioxide, no acidosis, and no change in pulmonary artery pressures, all of which is in direct contrast to the hypercapnia, acidosis, and increased pulmonary pressures observed during CO_2 insufflation [14]. Additionally, helium resulted in no change in heart rate, cardiac output, or arterial blood pressure, and no adverse effects such as arrhythmias, hypotension, or acid-base disturbances [23]. In twenty human patients undergoing laparoscopic cholecystectomy, there were no changes observed in hemodynamic variables, including arterial blood pressure, heart rate, or cardiac output with either the CO_2 or helium groups [4].

Helium as an insufflating gas displays many of the required properties, including inertness, availability, and safety. It has also been shown to eliminate the associated problems of hypercapnia [6]. The one major short-coming of helium is its relative insolubility in blood compared with CO_2, thus making the risk of death from the extremely infrequent complication of venous gas embolism (0.0016%–0.013%) [3] an ever present, albeit rare, reality. Overall, helium has the potential of becoming a clinically employed insufflating gas; however, more investigation is required.

Argon

In one pig study, argon as an insufflating gas produced an increased systemic vascular resistance index, a decreased stroke volume index, and a decreased cardiac index compared to a non-insufflated abdomen [5]. When compared to previously obtained data from CO_2 insufflation, argon was found to have a more significant depressant effect on hemodynamics than the previously studied CO_2 [5]. Further investigations will also be required to determine the effects of argon peritoneum. Unfortunately, this study utilized previous laboratory historical controls which limits the interpretation of this data [2].

Abdominal Wall Retractors

An alternative to gas insufflation of the abdomen is the employment of abdominal wall retractors. In animal studies, the hemodynamic changes produced by CO_2 insufflation of increased arterial pressure, increased heart rate, and increased cardiac output, were not observed in the mechanical retraction group [18, 22]. In one clinical study, although extensive hemodynamic measurements were not performed, central filling pressures and femoral vein pressures were lower in the mechanical lift group than in the CO_2-insufflation group, while heart rate and arterial blood pressures were similar in both groups [15]. Mechanical retraction seems an attractive alternative to CO_2 insufflation; but due to the physical limitation of the visual field, it is probably not technically applicable in all laparoscopic procedures.

Conclusions

There are many and varied hemodynamic effects seen during laparoscopic pneumoperitoneum. There are effects resultant from hypercapnia: opposing stimulation of catecholamine release and depression of myocardial function (Fig. 1). There are competing effects on the vascular system, with an increase in systemic vascular resistance produced by central vasoconstriction, but also with an

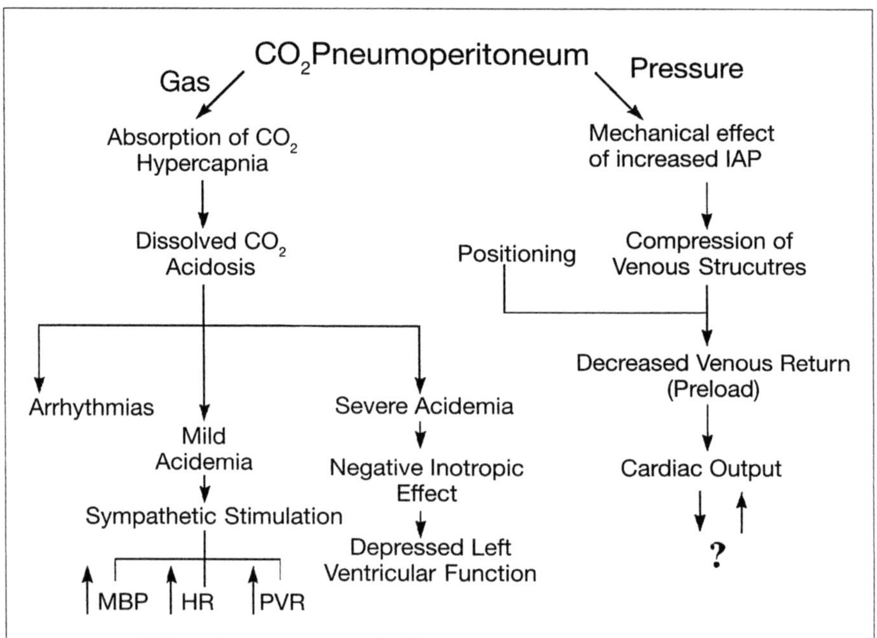

Fig. 1. Possible effects of gas and pressure of pneumoperitoneum. MBP, mean blood pressure; HR, heart rate; PVR, pulmonary venous pressure; IAP, intra-abdominal pressure

element of local vasodilatation [24]. The effect on preload is related to decreased venous return, an effect dependent on the patient's volume status and positioning. The effect on afterload is related to the increased systemic resistance resulting from both hypercapnia and vascular compression of the abdominal vessels. The resulting overall hemodynamic changes are dependent on the interaction of the above variables in patients with differing hemodynamic and pulmonary reserve and differing volume status. Insufflation of the abdomen has been generally shown to be safe [9]; it is, however, less well tolerated in certain high-risk patient populations [25, 30].

Summary

The hemodynamic changes seen with pneumoperitoneum are complex. As laparoscopy is performed in patients with less cardiac reserve, or in hemodynamically unstable situations, as in the critically ill patient in the intensive care unit, more invasive monitoring may be appropriate to ensure the safety of the patient.

References

1. Alexander GD, Brown EM (1969) Physiologic alterations during pelvic laparoscopy. Am J Obstet Gynecol 105:1078–1081
2. Andrus CH (1994) Invited commentary: Hemodynamic effects of argon pneumoperitoneum. Surg Endosc 8:322–323
3. Andrus CH, Wittgen CM, Naunheim KS (1994) Anesthetic and physiological changes during laparoscopy and thoracoscopy: the surgeon's view. Semin Laparosc Surg 1:228–240
4. Bongard FS, Pianim NA, Leighton TA, Dubecz S, Davis IP, Lippmann M, Klein S, Liu S (1993) Helium insufflation for laparoscopic operation. Surg Gynecol Obstet 177:140–146
5. Eisenhauer DM, Saunders CJ, Ho HS, Wolfe BM (1994) Hemodynamic effects of argon pneumoperitoneum. Surg Endosc 8:315–321
6. Fitzgerald SD, Andrus CH, Baudendistel LJ, Dahms TE, Kaminski DL (1992) Hypercarbia during carbon dioxide pneumoperitoneum. Am J Surg 163:186–190
7. Hashimoto S, Hashikura Y, Munakata Y, Kawasaki S, Makuuchi M, Hayashi K, Yanagisawa K, Numata M (1993) Changes in the cardiovascular and respiratory systems during laparoscopic cholecystectomy. J Laparoendosc Surg 3(6): 535–539
8. Ho HS, Saunders CJ, Gunther RA, Wolfe BM (1995) Effector of hemodynamics during laparoscopy: CO_2 absorption or intra-abdominal pressure. J Surg Res 59:497–503
9. Ishizaki Y, Bandai Y, Shimomura K, Abe H, Ohtomo Y, Idezuki Y (1992) Safe intra-abdominal pressure of carbon dioxide pneumoperitoneum during laparoscopic surgery. Surgery 114:549–554
10. Kashtan J, Green JF, Parsons EQ, Holcraft JW (1981) Hemodynamic effects of increased intra-abdominal pressure. J Surg Res 30:249–255
11. Kotzampassi K, Kapanidis N, Kazamias P, Eleftheriadis E (1993) Hemodynamic events in the peritoneal environment during pneumoperitoneum in dogs. Surg Endosc 7:494–499
12. Kubota K, Kajiura N, Teruya M, Ishihara T, Tsusima H, Ohta S, Nakao K, Arizono S (1993) Alterations in respiratory function and hemodynamics during laparoscopic cholecystectomy under pneumoperitoneum. Surg Endosc 7:500–504
13. Leighton T, Pianim M, Liu A, Kono M, Klein S, Bongard F (1992) Effectors of hypercarbia during experimental pneumoperitoneum. Am Surg 58:717–721

14. Leighton TA, Liu S, Bongard FS (1993) Comparative cardiopulmonary effects of carbon dioxide versus helium pneumoperitoneum. Surgery 113:527–531
15. Lindgren L, Koivusalo AM, Kellokumpu I (1995) Conventional pneumoperitoneum compared with abdominal wall lift for laparoscopic cholecystectomy. Br J Anaesth 75:567–572
16. Liu S, Leighton T, Davis I, Klein S, Lippmann M, Bongard F (1991) Prospective analysis of cardiopulmonary responses to laparoscopic cholecystectomy. J Laparoendosc Surg 1:241–246
17. Marshall RL, Jebson PJR, Kavie IT, Scott DB (1972) Circulatory effects of carbon dioxide insufflation of the peritoneal cavity for laparoscopy. Br J Anaesth 44:680–684
18. McDermott JP, Regan MC, Page R, Stokes MA, Barry D, Moriarty DC, Caushaj PF, Fitzpatrick JM, Gorey TF (1995) Cardiorespiratory effects of laparoscopy with and without gas insufflation. Arch Surg 130:984–988
19. McLaughlin JG, Scheeres DE, Dean RJ, Bonnell BW (1995) The adverse hemodynamic effects of laparoscopic cholcystectomy. Surg Endosc 9:121–124
20. Montalva M, Das B (1976) Carbon dioxide homeostasis during laparoscopy. South Med J 69:602–603
21. Motew M, Ivankovich AD, Bieniarz J, Albrecht RF, Zahed B, Scommegna A (1973) Cardiovascular effects and acid-base and blood gas changes during laparoscopy. Am J Obstet Gynecol 115:1002–1012
22. Rademaker BMP, Meyer DW, Bannenberg JJG, Klopper PJ, Kalkman CJ (1995) Laparoscopy without pneumoperitoneum. Surg Endosc 9:797–801
23. Rademaker BMP, Bannenberg JJG, Kalkman CJ, Meyer DW (1995) Effects of pneumoperitoneum with helium on hemodynamics and oxygen transport: a comparison with carbon dioxide. J Laparoendosc Surg 5:15–2
24. Rasmussen JP, Dauchot PJ, DePalma RG, Sorensen B, Regula G, Anton A, Gravenstein JS (1978) Cardiac function and hypercarbia. Arch Surg 113:1196–1200
25. Safran D, Sgambati S, Orlando R (1993) Laparoscopy in high-risk cardiac patients. Surg Gynecol Obstet 176:548–554
26. Scott DB, Julian DG (1972) Observations on cardiac arrhythmias during laparoscopy. BMJ 1:411–413
27. Smith I, Benzie RJ, Gordon NLM, Kelman GR, Swapp GH (1971) Cardiovascular effects of peritoneal insufflation of carbon dioxide for laparoscopy. BMJ 3:410–411
28. Van Den Bos GC, Drake AJ, Noble MI The effect of carbon dioxide upon myocardial contractile performance, blood flow and oxygen consumption. J Physiol 287:149–161
29. Williams MD, Murr PC (1993) Laparoscopic insufflation of the abdomen depresses cardiopulmonary function. Surg Endosc 7:12–16
30. Wittgen CM, Andrus CH, Fitzgerald SD, Baudendistel LJ, Dahms TE, Kaminski DL (1991) Analysis of the hemodynamic and ventilatory effects of laparoscopic cholecystectomy. Arch Surg 126:997–1001

10 Intra-abdominal Pressure, Intracranial Pressure, and Hemodynamics: A Central Nervous System-Regulated Response

R.J. ROSENTHAL, R.L. FRIEDMAN, and E.H. PHILLIPS

Introduction

Elevation in intra-abdominal pressure (IAP) can be classified as acute or chronic. The development of ascites from liver cirrhosis and portal hypertension, and the presence of retroperitoneal or intraperitoneal tumor masses are some of the more frequent examples of chronic elevation in IAP. The clinical significance of chronic elevations in IAP is related to the underlying pathology. Acute life-threatening changes are rarely observed. In contrast, acute elevations of intra-abdominal pressure have been shown to induce numerous serious hemodynamic, respiratory, and neurohormonal changes. The establishment of pneumoperitoneum in laparoscopic procedures or edema and hemoperitoneum in the abdominal compartment syndrome are the more frequent clinical settings of acute increase in IAP. The number of advanced laparoscopic procedures performed, combined with prolonged patient exposure to carbon dioxide (CO_2) has renewed interest in understanding the pathophysiologic effects of increased IAP.

In the past 30 years, many relevant papers have been published, though predominantly in the anesthesia, gynecology, and trauma literature. These reports describe the important hemodynamic and cardiorespiratory changes that occur in response to an increase in IAP. Thus far, no consensus has been reached in the explanation of some of these pathophysiologic changes. While some authors have shown evidence that a neurohormonal response mediated by chemoreceptors and osmoreceptors is involved, others have concluded that a mechanical effect is responsible for most of the changes [2–5]. We will try to elucidate this debate.

Intra-abdominal Pressure and Intracranial Pressure

In recent years, numerous investigators have reported in both animal and human studies that an increase in IAP produces an increase in intracranial pressure (ICP). These observations have been made for the most part during the creation of pneumoperitoneum in laparoscopic procedures or in the abdominal compartment syndrome seen in trauma patients. In 1994, in a large animal model, Josephs et al. [6] first observed that establishment of a pneumoperitoneum produces a significant increase in ICP. In his experiment at a pressure of 15 mmHg IAP, measurements of ICP were recorded at 30 min before, during, and after the creation of pneumoperitoneum. In addition, to evaluate the effects of IAP on a preexisting elevated ICP, an epidural balloon was inflated and this led to an increase in ICP. Then pneumoperitoneum was established. This resulted in a significant and immediate increase in ICP. They attributed these changes to a mechanical effect. The increase in IAP compresses the intra-abdominal large vessels, decreasing the outflow from the lumbar plexus. This results in an increased venous pressure in the vascular compartment of the spinal canal which, in turn, is transmitted to the intracranial vault, increasing ICP.

Based on Joseph's observations, our group performed a similar large animal model experiment; however, this time ICP was monitored at different increments of IAP and also in the Trendelenburg position [7]. In this study we used farm pigs with an average weight of 60 lb. Each animal served as its own control. The experiments performed in each animal were divided into two phases. Each phase was conducted with the animal in the supine (A) and Trendelenburg (B) position. During phase 1, animals had normal baseline ICP values; in phase II the baseline ICP values were artificially elevated by inflating a subdural balloon. ICP, mean arterial pressure (MAP), heart rate (HR), and arterial blood gases (ABG) were measured at various time points during each phase. Measurements were carried out in the supine (phases IA and IIA) and Trendelenburg position (phases IB and IIB) at 0, 8, 16, and 24 mmHg of IAP. Increases in IAP were achieved by creating pneumoperitoneum with CO_2 insufflation. The animals were mechanically ventilated with the aim of maintaining a baseline $PaCO_2$ of 35–45 mmHg. Anesthesia was sustained with an isofluorane/O_2 mixture (1.5%–5%). Continuous monitoring of ICP was performed with a transducer that was inserted intracranially and connected to a Camino V420 monitor. An additional burr hole was placed in the left prefrontal area, where a Foley catheter (8 F) was inserted into the subdural space. The catheter was used to artificially increase the ICP in phases IB and IIB. There was a significant and immediate linear increase in ICP at all levels of IAP. The Trendelenburg position further increased the ICP (Fig. 1) Another interesting observation was a parallel increase in mean blood pressure, but this change did not reach statistical significance. The cerebral perfusion pressures remained above critical levels throughout the experiment. Further investigations performed by our group showed the effects of the reverse-Trendelenburg position on ICP during acute elevations of IAP. As expected, there was a significant decrease in baseline values of ICP when compared to the supine and Trendelenburg positions. However, the establishment of IAP produced a significant increase in ICP (Fig. 2).

Both studies concurred that an increase in IAP produced an immediate effect on ICP. Similar findings are described by Irgau et al. in a patient with a cerebral glioma who had a laparoscopic cholecystectomy in which ICP monitoring was performed [8]. Since the rise in ICP observed in our animal studies was immediate and in both studies (those of Rosenthal and of Irgau) the $PaCO_2$ was maintained at or below 40 mmHg, it is not likely that an elevation in $PaCO_2$ occurred that could have been responsible for the increase in ICP. The insufflation of the abdominal cavity with CO_2 will produce an increase in $PaCO_2$, which, in turn, will produce a reflex vasodilatation of the cerebrovascular system that will further increase ICP. It has been demonstrated that it takes at least 10–15 min for the $PaCO_2$ to rise after pneumoperitoneum has been established [9,22]. In a recent publication, Schob et al. [10] demonstrated in a swine model that the establishment of pneumoperitoneum with nitrous oxide or helium produced a lesser increase in ICP than with CO_2. However, the fact that all three gases increased ICP supports the mechanical theory that other factors than arterial vasodilation produced by hypercapnia increases ICP.

In order to better understand the effects of increased IAP on the CNS, we postulate that the increase in ICP is mediated by two mechanisms. The first is an early mechanical or venous effect seen in the abdominal compartment syndrome, and with creation of pneumoperitoneum with or without CO_2 for laparoscopic procedures. The second is a late arterial or chemical effect seen mainly during laparoscopic procedures using CO_2 for pneumoperitoneum and with a prolonged compartment syndrome which results in hypercapnia (Fig. 10).

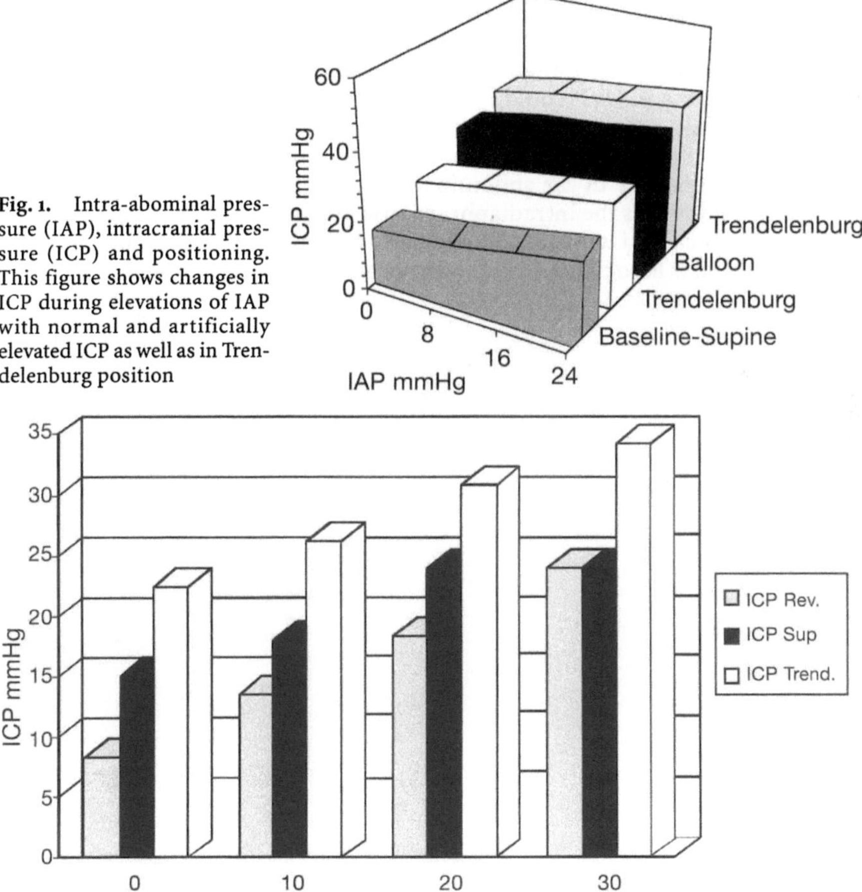

Fig. 1. Intra-abominal pressure (IAP), intracranial pressure (ICP) and positioning. This figure shows changes in ICP during elevations of IAP with normal and artificially elevated ICP as well as in Trendelenburg position

Fig. 2. Intra-abdominal pressure (IAP), intracranial pressure (ICP) and positioning. This figures shows changes in ICP during elevations of IAP in Trendelenburg (ICP Trend.) and Reverse Trendelenburg (ICP Rev.) position. Sup., supine

Early Stage (Venous or Mechanical Effect)

The increase in ICP during this stage has two components; an intra-abdominal and an intrathoracic. In the intra-abdominal effect, the establishment of an elevated IAP compresses the inferior vena cava (IVC) and produces an increase in central venous pressure (CVP) by reducing venous drainage from the CNS and lumbar plexus, thereby increasing the pressure in the CSF. Doppman et al. [12] showed in a dog model that the increase in IAP caused by fluids or gas in the abdominal cavity will produce a narrowing of the IVC at the level of the diaphragm. Rubinson et al. [13] came to similar conclusions in his studies. This caval obstruction disappeared when the IAP was released. Similar findings were described by Mullane et al. [14], and Ranninger et al. [15] in cirrhotic patients with ascites. In our study we were able to corroborate Doppman's observations. During pneumoperitoneum with IAP values at 0, 10, 20 and 30 mmHg, the IVC became narrowed at the level of the diaphragm (Figs. 3–6). The CVPs monitored above and below the diaphragm showed a simultaneous increase in pressure. Further variations in CVP could be observed in both regions based on animal positioning (Figs. 7, 8). It appears that it is not the increase in intra-abdominal pressure itself that compresses the large vessels of the abdomen, but rather that the increased pressure in the abdominal cavity displaces the diaphragm cranially which compresses the intradiaphragmatic portion of the IVC. This compression site was localized with cavography and exists above the liver and below the diaphragm and is associated with gradients across the affected segment.

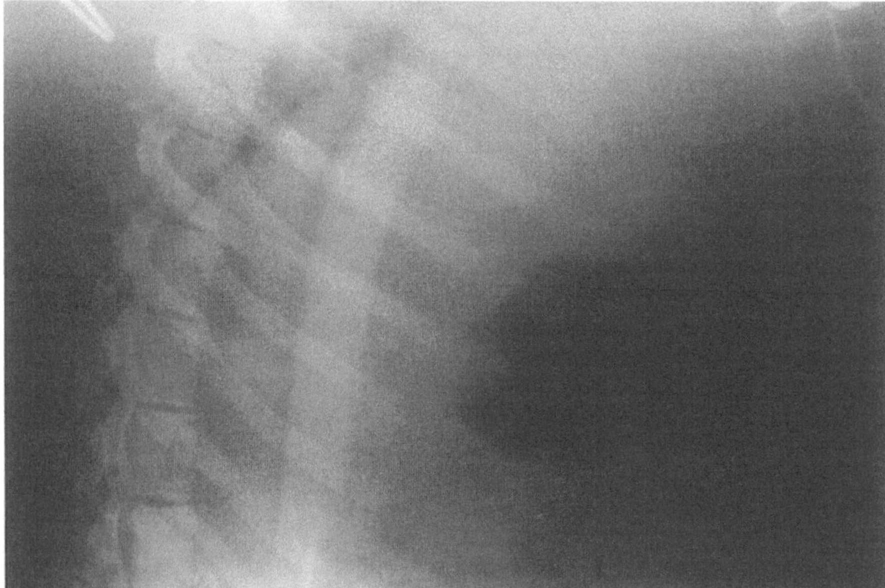

Fig. 3.   Cavogram. Diameter of the inferior vena cava at the level of the diaphragm without increased IAP

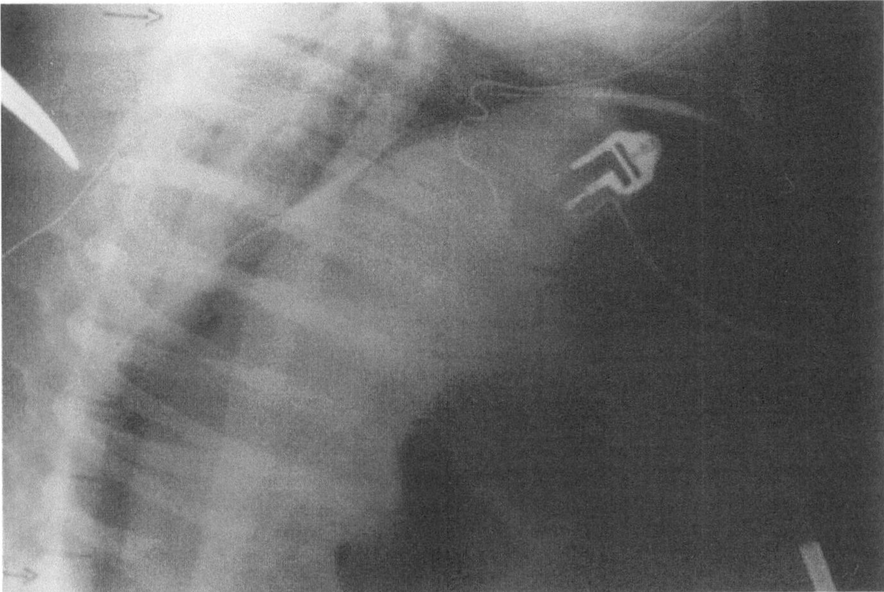

Fig. 4. Cavogram. Diameter of the inferior vena cava at the level of the diaphragm with IAP of 10 mmHg

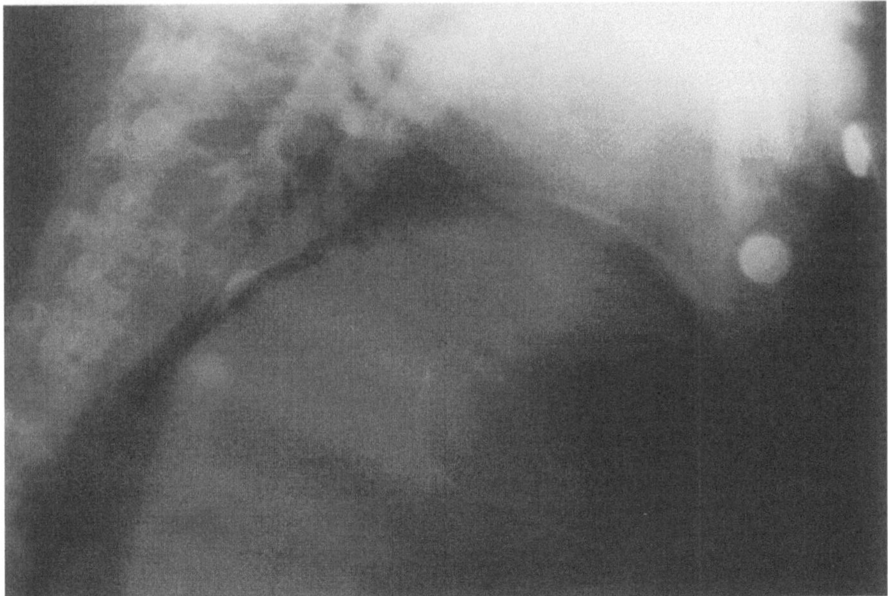

Fig. 5. Cavogram. Diameter of the inferior vena cava at the level of the diaphragm with IAP of 20 mmHg

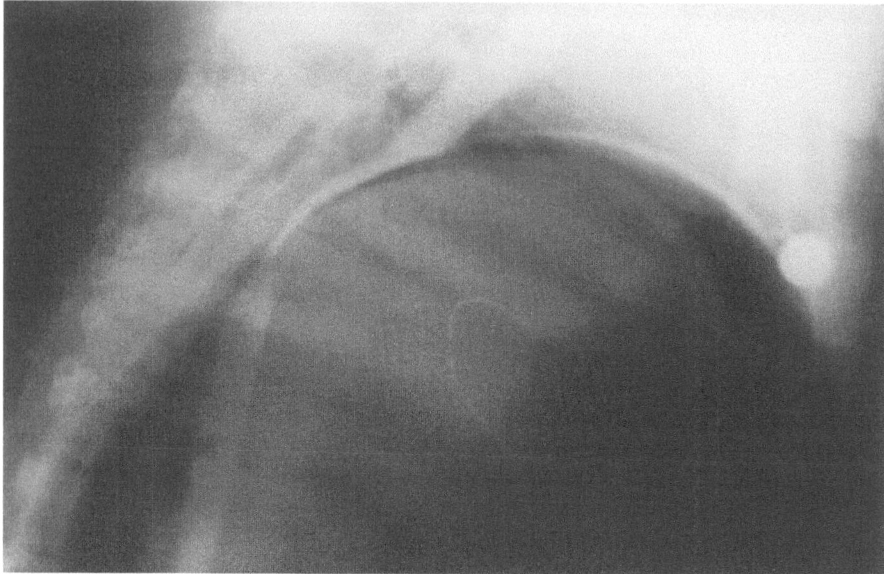

Fig. 6. Cavogram. Diameter of the inferior vena cava at the level of the diaphragm with IAP of 30 mmHg

The intrathoracic effect causing an increase in ICP correlates with the elevation in CVP above the diaphragm (Fig. 7). The cranial displacement of the diaphragm increases intrathoracic pressure by reducing the intrathoracic space and compressing the right atrium. This increases the cardiac filling pressure and the CVP in the superior vena cava (SVC) [40]. The intra-abdominal and intrathoracic components together decrease the venous drainage from the CNS, increasing the pressure in the sagittal sinus where the coroid plexus empties, thereby increasing ICP [11, 56]. In fact, Rubinson et al. observed that by increasing the intra-abdominal pressure there was a decrease in blood flow in the intrathoracic vena cava by 10%–18%, further corroborating our theory [13].

In a dog model, Luz et al. [40] showed that the combination of increased IAP and added positive end-expiratory pressure produces a significant decrease in cardiac output (CO) (decreased flow > decreased venous return > increased CVP) from 99 mmHg to 89 mmHg in the mean. They concluded that although the increase in intrathoracic pressure with a concomitant increase in CVP will decrease the risks of pulmonary embolism, the same effect precipitates serious hemodynamic problems related to decreased venous return and cardiac output (CO) [39]. The increase in ICP related to the increase in CVP can be explained by the Monroe-Kellie hypothesis. If one of the four compartments of the CNS (vascular, parenchyma, osseous, or CSF) expands rapidly, there is insufficient time for the other compartments to buffer those changes and ICP rises [16, 17]. This phenomenon was also seen in our study in which a significant increase in ICP was observed with low (8 mmHg) pressures of pneumoperitoneum and the animal in Trendelenburg position [23].

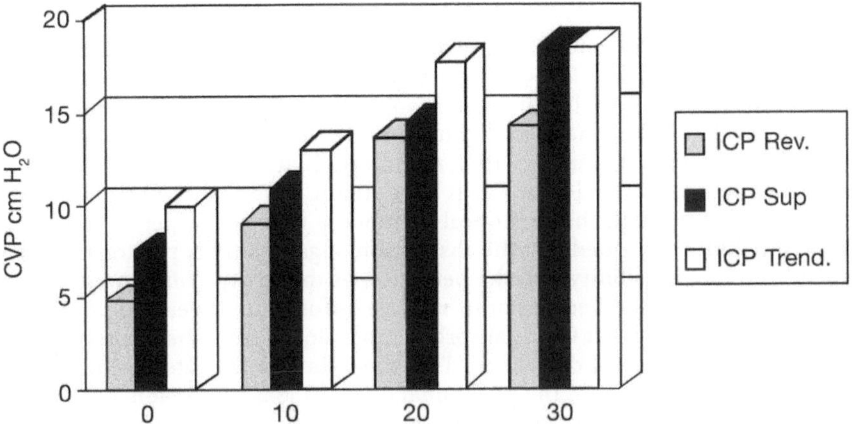

Fig. 7. Intra-abdominal pressure (IAP) and central venous pressure (CVP) above the diaphragm. This figures shows changes in CVP during elevations of IAP in Trendelenburg (CVP Trend.) and Reverse Trendelenburg (CVP Rev.) position. Sup., supine

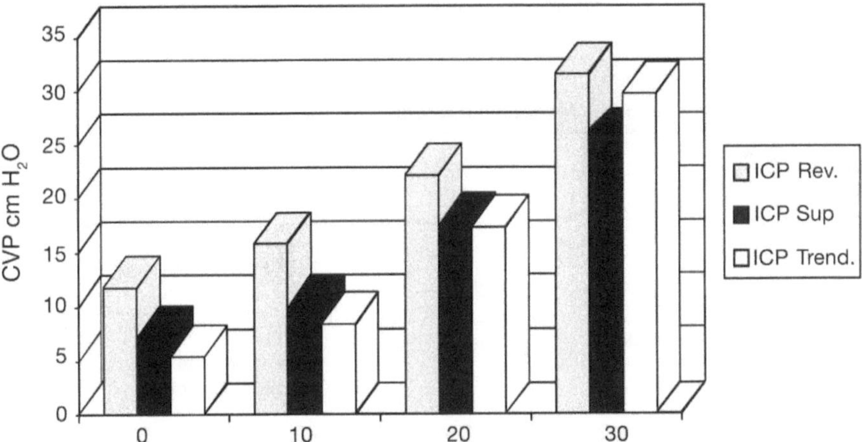

Fig. 8. Intra-abdominal pressure (IAP) and central venous pressure (CVP) below the diaphragm. This figures shows changes in CVP during elevations of IAP in Trendelenburg (CVP Trend.) and Reverse Trendelenburg (CVP Rev.) position. Sup., supine

Slagsvold et al. [18] demonstrated that when patients undergoing pneumoencephalography were placed in Trendelenburg position, there was a 20% higher incidence of retinal hemorrhage as compared to those that were placed in the supine position. He concluded that the reason for this side effect was mainly increased ICP due to decreased venous return.

Late Stage (Arterial or Chemical Effect)

In this stage the increase in ICP is mediated by hypercapnia which results from two distinct mechanisms (Fig. 9). The first mechanism involves the effects of CO_2 which is absorbed by simple diffusion through the peritoneal membrane into the preperitoneal capillary beds and cannot be removed with ventilation. This results in an increase in $PaCO_2$ with a reflex vasodilatation of the CNS vasculature which increases ICP [19, 20]. It is a fact that CO_2 is absorbed from the abdominal cavity through the peritoneal membrane into the preperitoneal capillaries [21]. Pilper described that the absorption of gas from the peritoneal cavity depends on its diffusibility and the perfusion of the cavity. Diffusion of CO_2 is unlikely to be impaired because of its relative diffusibility (twenty times that of air). He also reported that CO_2 is absorbed more slowly from the peritoneal cavity than from the pleural cavity [21]. This suggests that the rate limiting factor for absorption of CO_2 from the abdominal cavity is local perfusion, but surface area plays a role. In pneumoperitoneum, the sustained elevation in intra-abdominal pressure and increase in peripheral vascular resistance further restricts the blood perfusion of the preperitoneal capillary bed. Therefore, a delay may occur in the absorption of carbon dioxide from the abdominal cavity which delays the anticipated rise in $PaCO_2$ during the initial insufflation phase. Pilper also observed a significant elevation in $PaCO_2$ upon release of the intra-abdominal pressure [21]. The cranial excursion of the diaphragm due to the increase in IAP, combined

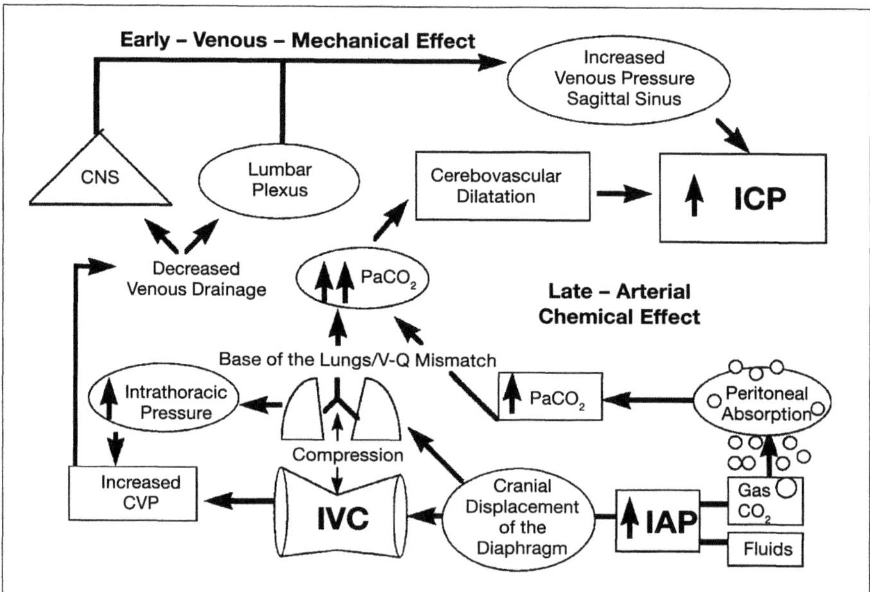

Fig. 9. Reasons for increased intracranial pressure (ICP) during acute elevations of intra-abdominal pressure (IAP). CNS, central nervous system; CVP, central venous pressure; IVC, inferior vena cava

with Trendelenburg position, compresses the lower lobes of the lungs, altering the ventilation perfusion ratio, which further increases the $PaCO_2$.

There is sufficient evidence in the literature supporting a direct effect of elevated $PaCO_2$ on ICP. In 1954, Westlake et al. [23] studied emphysematous patients with a high $PaCO_2$ and acute respiratory infections. They found the patients to have elevated cerebrospinal fluid (CSF) pressures. It was observed that these patients exhibited signs and symptoms of elevated ICP (headache, blurred vision, and papilledema), as described by Newton et al. [24]. Recently, Fuji et al. [25] concluded that the creation of CO_2 pneumoperitoneum in patients undergoing laparoscopic cholecystectomy produced hypercapnia and reflex vasodilatation of the CNS with increased flow through the middle cerebral artery. He showed a positive correlation between increased $PaCO_2$ and cerebral blood flow. The increased cerebral blood flow reflects a correspondingly large increase in total cerebral blood flow which in turn results in an increase in ICP, as stated by Monroe-Kellie. In contrast to Joseph's, Irgau's, and our study where an immediate increase in ICP was seen after the IAP was created, Fuji showed that cerebral blood flow increased 10 min after peritoneal insufflation parallel to the rise in $PaCO_2$. Likewise, 10 min after peritoneal deflation the blood flow and $PaCO_2$ returned to baseline values. These observations were confirmed by Liu et al. in a similar study [27].

Hemodynamic Response to Increased Intra-abdominal Pressure

Most of the adverse effects caused by an acute elevation in IAP on hemodynamics and on cardiorespiratory and renal function have been described in both the clinical and experimental literature and are also described in detail elsewhere in this book.

Mesenteric, Hepatic, and Abdominal Wall Blood Flow

Diebel et al. conducted numerous large animal studies which showed a graded and reproducible pattern of hemodynamic changes induced by increased IAP [28, 30]. They increased IAP with intraperitoneal instillation of Ringer's lactate and measured mesenteric arterial, hepatic arterial, portal, and abdominal wall blood flow. All splanchnic vascular beds, except the adrenal glands, showed an increase in vascular resistance with decreased blood flow to the affected organs. Similar observations were made by other authors in animal or human studies [31, 32].

Renal Blood Flow

Caldwell et al. showed in a large animal model that increased IAP produced by inflation of an intraperitoneal bag decreased renal blood flow and glomerular filtration rate and increased peripheral vascular resistance [33]. Harman et al. and Kashtan et al. came to the same conclusions [34, 35]. Smith et al. reported a case in which postoperative anuria was reversed by decompressive celiotomy.

Richards et al. [36] demonstrated a return of renal function following release of abdominal distention in patients requiring re-exploration for hemorrhage or abdominal distention. Possible mechanisms for the renal ischemia and anuria in these studies include direct parenchymal compression, caval or renal vein obstruction, compression of aortic or regional arterial supply, and neurohormonal dysfunction.

Central Venous Pressure, Mean Blood Pressure, and Peripheral Vascular Resistance

The previously mentioned studies found an increase in peripheral vascular resistance, central venous pressure (CVP), and mean blood pressure as signs of a sympathetic response to increased IAP.

Case Report

In 1995 Bloomfield et al. reported a patient with a head injury who had increased ICP secondary to acute abdominal compartment syndrome [37]. As the abdominal distention ensued, the patient had increased central venous and mean arterial pressure, as well as oliguria. Because of rising ICP, a decompressive celiotomy was performed. The patient's hemodynamics, cardiac, pulmonary, and renal function improved dramatically. The ICP declined and it was possible to withdraw inotropic support from the patient. The hemodynamic response to increased IAP and decompression has been previously described by other authors confronted with patients who had an abdominal compartment syndrome, ascites, or a prolonged laparoscopic procedure with CO_2 pneumoperitoneum [1, 38–44].

Hemodynamic Response to Increased Intracranial Pressure

Having demonstrated that increased IAP causes an increase in ICP, it is imperative to review the effects of ICP on hemodynamics. In 1881 Naunyn first described a pressor response where mean arterial pressure was stabilized at a level above that of a raised ICP [45]. This response was confirmed by Cushing in 1901 [46] and has since been called the Cushing reflex. The etiology and location of the receptors initiating the Cushing reflex have been identified by Hoff and Reis and are located in the lower brainstem [47]. They localized a cluster of adrenergic neurons (C1 area of the rostral ventrolateral medulla oblongata) in the brainstem reticular formation that act as the principal regulating area for resting, reflex, and behaviorally coupled control of arterial pressure [9]. The stimulus for this response originates in extreme cases of cerebral ischemia (Cushing or ischemic reflex), or in normal situations (physiologic circumstances) of increased ICP from simple distortion of the receptor cells in the C1 area of the medulla oblongata [48]. Most authors agree that the Cushing reflex is to prevent CNS ischemia by maintaining cerebral circulation in acute or chronic diseases with increased ICP [10]. This hemodynamic response is mediated by a sympathetic stimulus. These observations were confirmed by Brown [49] and others [50–53] who showed that there is an increase in venous tone following transient increases in ICP due to sympathetic discharge and release of catecholamines and vasopressin. The fact that the threshold for stimulating the receptive area ranges from 10–30 cm of H_2O, shows how sensitively the CNS reacts to changes in ICP. Furthermore, these distorting forces are sometimes generated by simple vascular pulsations.

Hemodynamic Parameters in the CNS Reaction

Studies performed in chimpanzees have shown that the hemodynamic response to changes in the CNS consists mainly of two steps [54]. The first step is an increase in CVP which represents mobilization of blood volume through venoconstriction. The second step shows an initial increase in CO and MAP, followed by an increase in total peripheral resistance (TPR) and a decrease in CO. Further studies by Doba and Reis [55] showed that this response could be elicited by different stimuli to the C1 area of the medulla oblongata. This stimuli included an insertion of an extradural balloon, local pressure to the exposed floor of the fourth ventricle, injecting CSF into the brainstem, or stereotactic electrical stimulation of the brainstem. Similar to earlier studies, all these stimuli resulted in a graded pattern of evoked cardiovascular activity consisting of increased central venous and mean arterial pressure, bradycardia, reduction in blood flow, and increased peripheral vascular resistance in the femoral, mesenteric, and renal arterial beds [8].

Neurons in the C1 area are integrated with a wide range of cardiovascular reflexes including arterial pressure. The C1 neurons respond to a number of neurotransmitters, many of which are restricted to local circuit neurons in the region. The C1 area neurons are also a target for several drugs which regulate arterial pressure including clonidine and B-blockers. It appears that the C1 area neurons of the rostral ventrolateral reticular nucleus function as one of the brainstem's most critical output systems for regulating arterial pressure [48].

Unifying Hypothesis

The reported experimental and clinical data have shown that increased IAP will produce a significant and immediate increase in ICP. Increased ICP produces similar hemodynamic responses to the ones elicited by increased IAP.

Based on these observations, we postulate that increased IAP caused by either air, fluids, or solids will displace the diaphragm cranially, which produces a narrowing of the infradiaphragmatic vena cava, increasing intrathoracic pressure and compression of the right atrium (Fig. 9).

These changes translate into a decrease in venous blood flow and an increase in CVP in the infradiaphragmatic and supradiaphragmatic vena cava, as well as an increase in right atrial filling pressures. The acutely increased CVP will increase resistance in venous drainage from the lumbar plexus, as well as the large veins of the CNS, and produce an acute expansion of the intracranial vascular compartment and sagittal sinus, with subsequent increase in ICP as stated by the Monroe-Kellie hypothesis (Fig. 9).

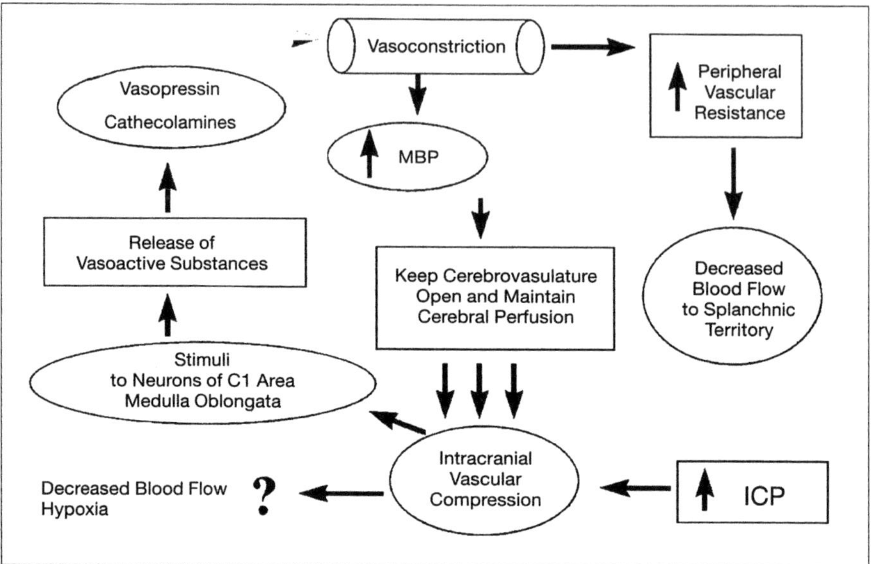

Fig. 10. Hemodynamic response to increased intracranial pressure (ICP) during acute elevations of intra-abdominal pressure. MBP, mean blood pressure

The increase in ICP will narrow the cerebrovascular system and produce a stimulus to the C1 neurons of the medulla oblongata which releases catecholamines and vasopressin (Fig. 10). The release of these vasoactive hormones produces venous and arterial vasoconstriction with increased mean blood pressure and increased peripheral vascular resistance to maintain adequate arterial cerebrovascular blood flow and cerebral perfusion. There is also mobilization of blood from intra-abdominal organs reflected in numerous studies as splanchic territory ischemia (Fig. 10). The delayed increase in ICP caused by the slow absorption of CO_2 from the abdominal cavity is augmented by a CNS-mediated increase in pulmonary vascular resistance. As mentioned earlier, the absorption of CO_2 from the abdominal cavity is regulated mainly by the diffusibility of gas into the peritoneal capillary bed, which in this case is constricted. This decreases diffusibility and absorption of CO_2 (Fig. 10). This hypothesis can be clinically applied in patients with acute elevations in IAP. Future studies may clarify if the same phenomenon occurs in chronic situations like ascites with liver cirrhosis or neoplasia.

References

1. Schein M, Wittmann DH, Aprahamian CC, Condon RE (1995) The abdominal compartment syndrome: the physiological and clinical consequences of elevated intra-abdominal pressure. J Am Coll Surg 180:745–753

2. Kashtan J, Green IF, Parsons EQ, Holcroft JW (1981) Hemodynamic effects of increased abdominal pressure. J Surg Res 30:249–255
3. Hodgson C, McClelland RMA, Newton JR (1970) Some effects of the peritoneal insufflation of carbon dioxide at laparoscopy. Anesthesiology 25(3):382–390
4. Motew M, Ivankovich AD, Bleniarz J, Albrecht RF, Zahed B, Scommenga A, Silverman B (1973) Cardiovascular effects and acid-base and gas changes during laparoscopy. Am J Obstet Gynecol 115(7):1002–1012
5. Kelman GR, Swapp GH, Smith I, Benzie RI, Gordon NLM (1972) Cardiac output and arterial blood gas tension during laparoscopy. Br J Anaesth 44:1155–1161
6. Josephs LG, Este McDonald JR, Birkett DH, Hirsch EF (1993) Diagnostic laparoscopy increases intracranial pressure. J Trauma 36(6):815–819
7. Rosenthal RI, Hiatt JA, Phillips EH, Hewitt W, Demetriou AA, Grode M (1997) Pneumoperiotneum related changes in intracranial pressure. Observations in a large animal model. Surg Endosc 11:376–380
8. Irgau I, Koyfman Y, Tikelis JL (1995) Elective intraoperative intracranial pressure monitoring during laparoscopic cholecystectomy. Arch Surg 130:1011–1013
9. Lewis DG, Ryder W, Burn K, Wheldon TJ, Tac-hi B (1972) Laparoscopy: an investigation during spontaneous ventilation with halothane. Br J Anesth 44:635–637
10. Schob OM, Allen DC, Benzel E, Curet MJ, Adams MS, Baldwin NG, Largiader F, Zucker KA (1996) A comparison of the pathophysiologic effects of carbon dioxide, nitrous oxide and helium pneumoperitoneum on intracranial pressure. Am J Surg 172:248–253
11. lmilhorat TH (1975) The third circulation revisited. J Neurosurg 42:628–645
12. Doppman J, Rubinson RM, Rockoff SD, Vasko JS, Shapiro R, Morrow AG (1966) Mechanism of obstruction of the infradiaphragmatic portion of the inferior vena cava in the presence of increased intra-abdominal pressure. Invest Radiol 1:37–53
13. Rubinson RM, Vasko JS, Doppman L, McCrow AG (1967) Inferior vena caval obstruction from increased intra-abdominal pressure. Arch Surg 94:766–770
14. Mullane JF, Gliedman ML (1966) Elevation of the pressure in the abdominal inferior vena cava as a cause of a hepatorenal syndrome. Surgery 59(6):1135–1146
15. Ranninger K, Switz DM (1965) Local obstruction of the inferior vena cava by massive ascites. Am J Roentgen 93:935–940
16. Spencer W, Horsely V (1892) On the changes produced in the circulation and respiration by increase of the intracranial pressure or tension. Philos Trans 182:201–254
17. Sullivan HG, Miller JD, Becker DP (1977) The physiological basis of intracranial pressure change with progressive epidural brain compression. J Neurosurg 47:532–534
18. Slagsvold JE (1977) Retinal hemorrhage as a complication of gas enceophalography and gas myelography. Prospective study using oxygen gas with a discussion of pathogenic mechanisms. J Neurol Neurosurg Psychiatry 20:1049–1052
19. Cullen LK, Steffey EP, Bailey CS, Kortz G, Da Silva VJ, Curiel J, Belhorn RW, Wollner MJ, Elliot AR, Jarvis KA (1990) Effect of high $PaCO_2$ and time on cerebrospinal fluid and intraocular pressure in halothane anesthetized horses. Am J Vet Res 51(2):300–304
20. Hargreaves DM (1990) Hypercapnia and raised cerebrospinal fluid pressure. Anesthesia 45(12):7–12
21. Pilper J (1965) Physiological equilibrium of gas cavities in the body. In: Feen WO, Rahn M (eds) Respiration, vol 2., pp 1025–1027 (Handbook of physiology, sect 3)
22. Hogdson C, McClelland AMA, Newton JR. (1970). Some effects of the peritoneal insufflation of carbon dioxide at laparoscopy . Anesthesia 25:382–390
23. Westlake EK, Kaye M (1954) Raised intracranial pressure in emphysema. BMJ 1:302–304
24. Newton DAG, Bone I (1979) Papilloedema and optic atrophy in chronic hypercapnia. Br J Dis Chest 73:399–404
25. Fujii Y, Tanaka H, Tsurukoa S, Toyooka H, Amaha K (1994) Middle Cerebral arterial blood flow velocity increases during laparoscopic cholecystectomy. Anesth Analg 78:80–83
26. Hansen N, Stonestreet B, Rosenkrantz T (1983) Validity of Doppler measurements of anterior cerebral artery blood flow velocity; correlation with cerebral blood flow in piglets. Pediatrics 72:526–531
27. Liu SY, Leighton T, Davis I (1991) Prospective analysis of cardiopulmonary responses to laparoscopic cholecystectomy. Laparoendosc Surg 1:241–246
28. Diebel LN, Saxe J, Dulchavsky S (1992) Effect of intra-abdominal pressure on abdominal wall blood flow. Am Surg 9: 573–576

29. Diebel LN, Wilson ME, Dulchavsky SA, Saxe J (1992) Effect of increased intra-abdominal pressure on hepatic arterial, portal venous and hepatic microcirculatory blood flow. J Trauma 33(2):279–283

30. Diebel LN, Dulchavsky SA, Wilson ME (1992) Effect of increased intra-abdominal pressure on mesenteric arterial and intestinal mucosal blood flow. J Trauma 33(1):45–49

31. Shimizu M, Yohizu H, Hatori N, Haga Y, Okuda E, Uriuda Y, Tanaka S (1990) Acute effect of intra-abdominal pressure on liver and systemic circulation. Vasc Surg 24:677–682

32. Eleftheriadis E, Kotzampassi K, Papanotas K, Heliadis N, Sarris K (1996) Gut ischemia, oxidative stress and bacterial translocation in elevated abdominal pressure. World J Surg 20:11–16

33. Caldwell CB, Ricotta JJ (1987) Changes in visceral blood flow with elevated intra-abdominal pressure. J Surg Res 43:14–20

34. Harman PK, Kron IL, Mc Lachlan HD (1982) Elevated intra-abdominal pressure and renal function. Ann Surg 196:594–596

35. Kashtan J, Green JF, Parsons EQ (1981) Hemodynamic effects of increased abdominal pressure. J Surg Res 30:249

36. Richards WO, Scovill W, Shin B (1983) Acute renal failure associated with increased intra-abdominal pressure. Ann Surg 97:183–187

37. Bloomfield GL, Dalton JM, Sugerman HJ, Ridings PC, DeMaria EJ, Bullock R (1995) Treatment of increasing intracranial pressure secondary to the acute abdominal compartment syndrome in a patient with combined abdominal and head trauma. J Trauma 39(6):1168–1170

38. Hashimoto S, Hashikura Y, Munakata Y, Kawasaki S, Makuuchi M, Hayashi K, Yanagisawa K, Numata M (1993) Changes in the cardiovascular and respiratory systems during laparoscopic cholecystectomy. J Laparoendosc Surg 3(6):535–539

39. Bradley SE, Bradley GP (1947) The effect of increased intra-abdominal pressure on renal function in man. J Clin Invest 26(2):1010–1022

40. Luz CM, Polarz H, Bohrer R, Hundt G, Dorsam J, Martin E (1994) Hemodynamic and respiratory effects of pneumoperitoneum and PEEP during laparoscopic pelvic lymphadenectomy in dogs. Surg Endosc 8:25–27

41. Ivankovich AD, Miletich DJ, Albrecht DR, Heyman HJ, Bonnet RF (1975) Cardiovascular effects of intraperitoneal insuflation with carbondioxide and nitrous oxide in the dog. Anesthesiology 42:281–287

42. Ho HS, Gunther RA, Wolfe BM (1992) Intraperitoneal carbon dioxide insufflation and cardiopulmonary functions. Arch Surg 127:928–933

43. Smith I, Benzie RJ, Gordon NLM, Kelman GR, Swapp GH (1971) Cardiovascular effects of peritoneal insufflation of carbon dioxide for laparoscopy. BMJ 14:410–411

44. Thorington JM, Schmidt CF (1923) A study of urinary output and blood pressure changes resulting in experimental ascites. Am J Med Sci 165(2):880–890

45. Naunyn B, Schreiber J (1881). J Arch Exper Path Pharmakol 14:1

46. Cushing H (1901). John Hopkins Med J 12:290–293

47. Hoff JT, Reis DJ (1970) Localization of regions mediating the Cushing response in CNS of cat. Arch Neurol 23:228–240

48. Reis DJ, Ruggiero DA, Morrison SF (1989) The C1 area of the rostral ventrolateral medulla oblongata. A critical brainstem region for control of resting and reflex integration of arterial pressure. AJR 2:363–374

49. Brown FK (1956) Cardiovascular effects of acutely raised intracranial pressure. Am J Physiol 185:510–514

50. Guyton AC (1991) Nervous regulation of the circulation and rapid control of arterial pressure. In: Guyton AC (ed): Physiology, 8th edn. Saunders, Philadelphia, pp 202–203

51. Le Roith D, Bark H, Nyksa M, Glick SM (1982) The effect of abdominal pressure on plasma antidiuretic, hormone levels in the dog. J Surg Res 32:65–69

52. Melville RJ, Frizis HI, Forsling ML, Le Quesne LP (1985) The stimulus of vasopressin release during laparoscopy. Surg Gynecol Obstet 161:253–256

53. Punnonen R, Vinamaki O (1982) Vasopressin release during laparoscopy. Lancet 1:175–176

54. Ducker TB, Simmons RL, Anderson RW, Kempe LG (1968) Hemodynamic cardiovascular response to raised intracranial pressure. Med Ann Columbia 37(10):523–526

55. Doba N, Reis DJ (1972) Localization within the brainstem of a receptive area mediating the pressor response to increased intracranial pressure (The Cushing response). Brain Res 47:487–491

56. Langfitt TW, Weinstein JD, Kassell NF, Gagliardi LJ (1964) Transmission of increased intracranial pressure within the supratentorial space. J Neurosurg 21:998–1005

11 Neurohormonal Response to Laparoscopy and Acute Rise in Intra-abdominal Pressure

C. CORWIN, A.J. FABREGA, and C. SCOTT-CONNER

Introduction

The clinical observation that the laparoscopic surgical approach lessens postoperative pain and shortens hospital stay [1, 2] when compared to open surgery, might lead one to postulate that laparoscopy is accompanied by a diminished postoperative physiologic stress response. Indeed, the very term "minimally invasive surgery" indirectly suggests this possibility. However, it is not yet clear that laparoscopy lessens the complex neurohormonal stress response which accompanies conventional surgery. There is an increasing body of research on the physiological changes which occur with pneumoperitoneum, as well as a growth of data on the related condition of an acute rise in intra-abdominal pressure and the abdominal compartment syndrome (ACS) [3–9].

This chapter will highlight the neurohormonal changes which occur during surgery and review the current research which has begun to delineate the neurohormonal response to both an acute rise in intra-abdominal pressure and the iatrogenic pneumoperitoneum. Finally, the available studies which compare the stress response to laparoscopic versus open cholecystectomy will be summarized.

Overview of the Neurohormonal Stress Response to Injury

To understand the response to pneumoperitoneum a brief overview of the neurohormonal stress response is in order (Fig. 1). The normal body responds to injury through a series of complex neural and hormonally mediated changes termed the neurohormonal stress response. These changes attempt to restore an injured organism to a normal state of homeostasis and health. Injury may take the form of tissue destruction, as in major trauma or surgery, or massive hemorrhage and infection. The changes which occur during major trauma and hemorrhage are quite dramatic. The changes which occur during elective surgical procedures (where measures are deliberately taken to minimize stress) may be more subtle, yet nonetheless scientifically revealing and clinically important.

Tissue injury directly stimulates the sensory (afferent) nervous system. It also causes mediators of inflammation (i.e., histamine, kinins, prostaglandins, peptides, interleukins, and components of the complement system) to accumulate in and stimulate the region of injury. Fibers carrying the afferent stimulus travel within the spinothalamic tracts in the spinal cord to converge in the medulla and pons [10]. Afferent input is integrated and processed in the hypo-

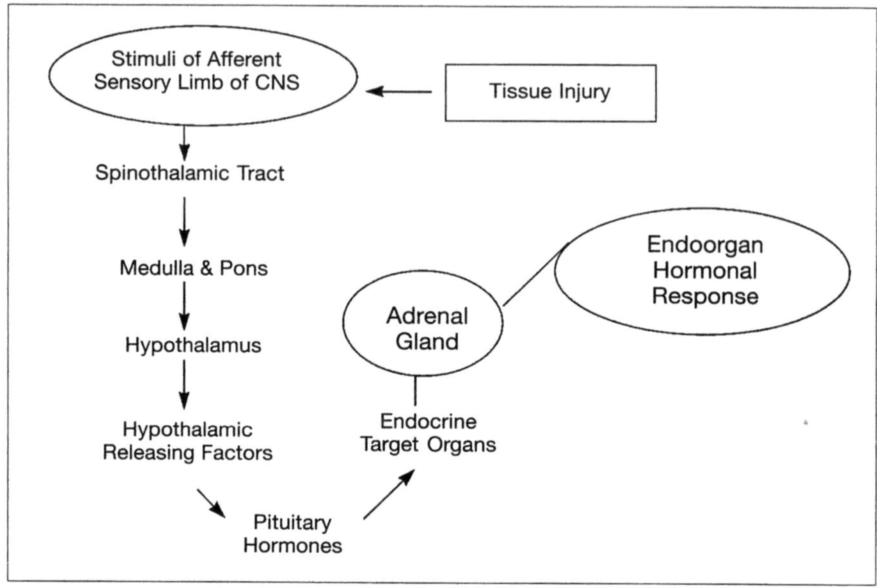

Fig. 1. The neurohormonal stress response

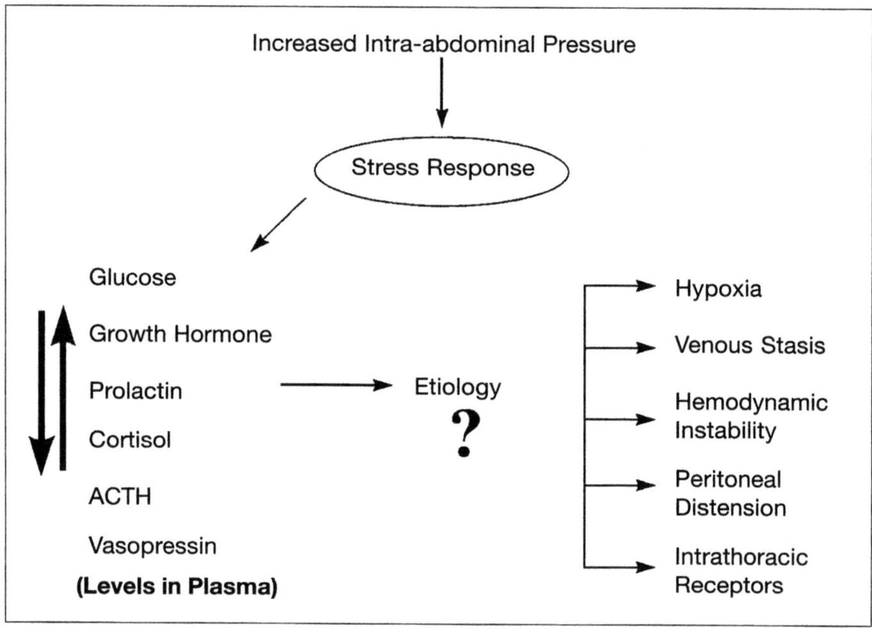

Fig. 2. Increased intra-abdominal pressure and the neurohormonal stress response. ACTH, adrenocorticotropic hormone

thalamus and hypothalamic releasing factors are secreted. Pituitary hormones then transmit the neural stimulus to the endocrine target organs, creating an end-organ hormonal response. Activation of the hypothalamic-pituitary-adrenal axis increases secretion of catabolic hormones (i.e., cortisol, glucagon, and catecholamines), and generally inhibits secretion of anabolic hormones. These hormonal changes result in a measurable "neurohormonal stress response," which is characterized by substrate mobilization and, ultimately, a catabolic state with negative nitrogen balance (Fig. 2).

Afferent Limb

The initiator mechanism of the hormonal response is predominantly mediated through neurogenic stimuli from the surgical area [11]. The role of afferent neurogenic stimuli from the site of surgery to the hypothalamus became evident during early studies in which epidural analgesia was used to block the afferent stimuli from the site of surgery. Such studies demonstrated, to varying degrees, a diminished hormonal response under epidural analgesia, including decreased secretion of cortisol, growth hormone, and prolactin [12–14].

Hypothalamus

Antidiuretic hormone (ADH), also known as vasopressin, is synthesized by the paraventricular and supraoptic nuclei of the hypothalamus and secreted as part of neurophysin I. Neurophysin I is then cleaved into ADH and neurophysin in the posterior pituitary. ADH binds to the distal convoluted tubules in the kidney where it increases the permeability of the tubular epithelium to water. This results in a shift of water into the hyperosmolar medullary interstitium of the kidney. The kidney then produces a decreased volume of more concentrated urine resulting in water and salt retention and a decrease in plasma osmolality. ADH secretion responds to changes in both increased plasma osmolality and decreased plasma volume [15]. The relationship of ADH secretion to surgical stress has been of research interest for the past 40 years when the bioassay used to measure ADH first became available [16–19]. A decrease in plasma volume associated with major surgery or trauma increases ADH secretion and water retention. It has also been hypothesized that a major stimulus to the secretion of ADH during surgery is the neuronal impulse arising from the surgical site. Several studies have been published which attempt to delineate the roles of neuronal impulses arising from the surgical site and plasma volume changes in the secretion of ADH during surgical stress [20].

Pituitary Gland

Surgical stress has been shown to influence the secretion of various pituitary hormones [12, 21–23]. Adrenocorticotropic hormone (ACTH) is secreted by the anterior pituitary gland in response to corticotropin-releasing factor (CRF) from the hypothalamus. Receptors in the adrenal cortex bind ACTH, stimulating the secretion of cortisol and other steroid precursors. ACTH increases aldosterone secretion by the adrenal cortex. Both cortisol and aldosterone promote sodium resorption in the proximal renal tubule resulting in intravascular volume expansion. Cortisol also inhibits the secretion of various cytokines and other pro-inflammatory mediators, potentially inhibiting the inflammatory response. ACTH has been shown to increase with surgical stress [21, 24, 25].

Growth hormone is secreted by the anterior pituitary gland and is under both stimulatory and inhibitory control by hypothalamic releasing factors. Similar to ACTH, growth hormone secretion has a normal circadian rhythm and increases with stress. Exercise, protein depletion, glucagon, and L-dopa also stimulate growth hormone secretion. Growth hormone promotes the mobilization of glycogen stores and protein synthesis, both of which are crucial for perioperative events such as wound healing. Hyperglycemia suppresses the secretion of growth hormone.

Prolactin is secreted by the anterior pituitary gland. Prolactin secretion is under inhibitory control by dopamine, which is released by the hypothalamus. Prolactin stimulates breast development and lactation in females and testosterone secretion in males. Prolactin secretion increases during major surgery. General anesthesia in itself is a major stimulus for prolactin increase [12]. Prolactin has also been shown to increase during experimental surgery without anesthesia [22].

Endocrine Target Organs

Adrenal Gland

The adrenal gland has a cortex which produces steroid hormones and a medulla which produces catecholamines. Cortisol is synthesized from cholesterol in the zona fasciculata of the adrenal cortex. Cortisol increases after injury due to both an increase in ACTH secretion and an increase in adrenal sensitivity to ACTH. Cortisol stimulates gluconeogenesis and increased deposition of liver glycogen. Injury is typically associated with a hyperglycemic response. Aldosterone is the primary mineralocorticoid secreted by the zona glomerulosa of the adrenal cortex. Through proximal resorption of sodium and chloride by the renal tubules and distal resorption of sodium, aldosterone causes sodium retention and, indirectly, water retention. Aldosterone release is primarily under control of the renin-angiotensin system. Hypovolemia (which occurs with major surgery) is sensed by the juxtaglomerular complex in the kidney and activates the renin–angiotensin system, leading to an increase in angiotensin II and aldosterone release. Aldosterone release is also stimulated by hyperkalemia and ACTH.

The sympathoadrenal system is considered the prototype neuroendocrine system. Epinephrine is secreted by the adrenal medulla and travels through the circulation to the target cells. Norepinephrine is released from axon terminals of sympathetic postganglionic neurons and delivered directly to the innervated target cells. Various neural triggers associated with injury and surgery cause an increase in catecholamine secretion. Catecholamine release results in a wide variety of physiologic alterations, including hemodynamic changes (increase in blood pressure) and metabolic reactions (hyperglycemia) [26].

Renin–Angiotensin System

Juxtaglomerular Cells of the Kidney

Renin is secreted by the juxtaglomerular cells of the kidney when decreased renal blood flow is sensed. The juxtaglomerular cells also secrete renin in response to sympathetic stimulation. Renin enzymatically cleaves angiotensinogen, causing the release of angiotensin I. A converting enzyme, present within the pulmonary microvasculature, converts angiotensin I to angiotensin II. Angiotensin II is a potent vasoconstrictor and also potentiates the release of other mediators of the neuroendocrine response, such as aldosterone, catecholamines, ADH, and ACTH. ADH secretion and hyperkalemia are both inhibitory controls of renin secretion. The significance of surgery and pneumoperitoneum is described in detail in Chap. 7.

Pancreas

Hypoglycemia is the primary stimulus for glucagon release from the alpha cells of the pancreatic islets. Glucagon stimulates gluconeogenesis directly, as well as indirectly by causing an increase in free fatty acids. Glucagon promotes glycogenolysis by increasing levels of cyclic adenosine monophosphate (cAMP). Thus glucagon causes hyperglycemia as a result of both glycogenolysis and gluconeogenesis. Glucagon secretion is also increased during injury. This response is augmented by a-adrenergic stimulation and possibly by catecholamine release. Sympathetic and parasympathetic pathways, by way of the hypothalamus, may also be involved in the stimulation of glucagon secretion.

The release of insulin from the beta cells of the pancreatic islets is stimulated by hyperglycemia and parasympathetic activity. Normally, the hyperglycemia which accompanies injury results in some increase in insulin release; however, circulating catecholamines and a-adrenergic activity moderate this response and prevent insulin from reaching very high levels under stressful conditions. This, in combination with insulin resistance, allows the variable degrees of hyperglycemia normally seen under conditions of stress or injury [27].

Neurohormonal Changes During an Acute Increase in Intra-Abdominal Pressure and Laparoscopic Pneumoperitoneum

The effect of increased abdominal pressure on the neurohormonal stress response is inherently difficult to measure. The various studies and reviews of the physiological changes which occur during the abdominal compartment syndrome primarily focus on the hemodynamic and respiratory consequences of an acute rise in intra-abdominal pressure. It was not until the expansion in laparoscopic surgery that more data regarding hormonal changes under the condition of increased abdominal pressure became available. While several animal models have been utilized, the laparoscopic iatrogenic pneumoperitoneum is the most relevant clinical model for studying the hormonal changes which occur during conditions of increased intra-abdominal pressure. Available clinical studies will be summarized here.

Acute Rise in Intra-Abdominal Pressure

Antidiuretic Hmormone

The relationship between ADH secretion and increased intra-abdominal pressure has been of interest for many years. The actual mechanism for the relationship between increased abdominal pressure and ADH secretion is not well understood. Studies using various models of increased abdominal pressure, including the cirrhotic patient with tense ascites, as well as laparoscopic pneumoperitoneum, have attempted to document the ADH response to increased intra-abdominal pressure and better define the underlying mechanism of this response.

Two decades ago, Husain et al. [28] demonstrated an increase in ADH release after manual abdominal compression in rats. This increase was not reproducible by other forms of physical or emotional stress (i.e., noise, forced activity, light, ether, anesthesia). The authors postulated that the stimulus for ADH release was either hypoxia [29] or a sudden change in circulating blood volume due to trapping of blood in the lower body. Le Roith et al. [30] subsequently showed that abdominal pressure (80 mmHg) applied to anesthetized dogs resulted in an elevation of ADH levels to greater than twice basal levels. Cardiac output fell concomitant with a rise in ADH after applied abdominal pressure and the authors proposed that altered hemodynamics were the stimulus for ADH release. This theory was supported when the fall in cardiac output and the elevation in ADH was prevented by volume expansion with dextran.

Subsequent human studies confirmed the finding of increased ADH secretion in animals with elevated intra-abdominal pressure. Punnonen and Viinamaki [31] studied 12 female patients undergoing laparoscopy and demonstrated that plasma ADH concentration was significantly ($p < 0.05$) higher at the end of the pneumoperitoneum insufflation phase. As no patient experienced respiratory or hemodynamic compromise during the laparoscopy, the authors concluded that increased intra-abdominal pressure and peritoneal distention had a direct stimulating effect on ADH release.

In an attempt to confirm the relationship between increased intra-abdominal pressure and elevated ADH levels in humans, Melville et al. performed a subsequent study on 11 women undergoing laparoscopy for fertility related surgery [32]. During all 11 procedures, the maximum intra-abdominal pressure obtained was 45 mmHg (very high pressures by today's standards). The authors demonstrated a prompt rise ($p < 0.01$) and fall in ADH levels associated with the rise and fall in intra-abdominal pressure with pneumoperitoneum. A close temporal relationship between the parallel changes in intra-abdominal pressure and ADH levels was evident. The rise in ADH was not associated with the induction of anesthesia, nor accounted for by a fall in mean blood pressure or changes in serum osmolality. The authors suggested that the relationship between intra-abdominal pressure and ADH secretion is mediated by the trapping of blood in the lower part of the body and decreased venous return to the heart which is sensed by intrathoracic blood volume receptors located in the left atrium.

Herruzo et al. studied 47 patients with varied diagnoses undergoing diagnostic laparoscopy, and documented a significant increase in ADH [33]. The increased ADH secretion was independent of the presence of underlying liver disease and method of anesthesia (general vs local). Because mean blood pressure, osmolality, and oxygenation remained constant during laparoscopy, the increase in ADH secretion could not be attributed to decreased plasma volume, increased osmolality or hypoxia. A significant increase in right atrial venous pressures correlated with elevated ADH levels, suggesting that the ADH response could be due to a decrease in the left atrial transmural pressure gradient. This gradient has been shown to be a stimulus for ADH release in other studies [34].

Most recently, Volz et al. performed a study of the pathophysiologic features of pneumoperitoneum during laparoscopy in a swine model [35]. In this study, animals were divided into five groups: six animals with carbon dioxide and intra-abdominal pressure of 14 mmHg, six animals with air and intra-abdominal pressure of 14 mmHg, five animals with carbon dioxide and intra-abdominal pressure of 18 mmHg, five animals with air and intra-abdominal pressure of 18 mmHg, and three animals without pneumoperitoneum. In contrast to the previously reviewed studies, the authors failed to establish a difference in plasma ADH levels among any of the groups. This illustrates a general problem; while most data reveal a stimulatory effect of increased intra-abdominal pressure on ADH secretion, this response has not always been reproducible. To date, the mechanism of the pronounced ADH response to laparoscopy remains largely undefined. Whether the rise in ADH is secondary to hemodynamic, mechanical, or nociceptive stimulation is still a matter of considerable controversy [36]. The clinical significance of elevated ADH levels with an increase in intra-abdominal pressure during surgical pneumoperitoneum also remains unclear. It is possible that elevated levels of ADH during laparoscopy explains the well described, but poorly studied, phenomenon of oliguria which occurs during both abdominal compartment syndrome and iatrogenic pneumoperitoneum [37].

Laparoscopy and the Iatrogenic Pneumoperitoneum

Anterior Pituitary–Adrenocortical–Adrenomedullary Axis and Glucose Metabolism

Knowledge of the anterior pituitary-adrenocortical response to an acute rise in intra-abdominal pressure remains limited. The majority of information has been obtained through studies which compare the hormonal stress response accom-

Table 1. Neurohormonal stress response to surgery: laparoscopy versus conventional surgery

Reference	Procedure	ADH	Renin	Aldo-sterone	ACTH	Cortisol	Catecho-lamines	GH	Pro-lactin	Glucose	Insulin	Glucagon
Punnonen [31]	L	↑										
Melville [32]	L	↑										
Herruzo [33]	L	↑										
Voltz [35]	L	↔										
Mansour [25]	LC				↑↑	↑↑					↔	↔
	OC				↑	↑					↔	↔
Cooper [39]	LC					↑		↑	↑	↑		
Milheiro [45]	LC		↑			↑						
	OC		↑			↑						
Deuss [21]	LC				↑			↑	↑			
	OC				↑			↔	↑			
Targarona [46]	LC				↑	↑		↑			↑	↑
	OC				↑	↑		↑			↑	↑
O'Leary [47]	LC		↑	↑	↑	↑		↑	↑			
Ortega [48]	LC	↑↑			↑	↑	↑			↑↑[a]	↑	↑
	OC	↑			↑	↑	↑			↑	↑↑[b]	↑↑[b]

ADH, antidiuretic hormone; ACTH, adrenocorticotropic hormone; GH, growth hormone; L, laparoscopy only; LC, laparoscopic cholecystectomy; OC, open cholecystectomy.
↑ Elevated;
↔ unchanged.
[a] Intraoperative.
[b] Postoperative.

panying laparoscopic cholecystectomy and the iatrogenic pneumoperitoneum to that which accompanies open cholecystectomy. Cholecystectomy has been the surgical model for most recent studies as cholecystectomy is one of the most frequently performed operations in general surgery [38]. It is well established and relatively noncontroversial that laparoscopy is associated with a stress response in the pituitary–adrenocortical axis [39]. However, whether the magnitude of this stress response is attenuated when compared to that generated by the open surgical approach remains a matter of significant controversy. Some studies demonstrate a decrease in the hormonal stress response [40], while others demonstrate an increase in certain catabolic stress related hormones [41]. Efforts to resolve this debate have stimulated much of the recent research on the stress response to laparoscopic surgery. While most of the recent data do not allow one to reach concrete conclusions regarding the pituitary-adrenal response to increased intra-abdominal pressure, they do provide some insight into the hormonal response to laparoscopy and the iatrogenic pneumoperitoneum. The studies to date are summarized in Table 1 and will be briefly discussed here.

Mansour et al. [25] compared the hormonal stress markers, ACTH, cortisol, insulin, and glucagon, measured prior to and for the first 3 postoperative days, in pigs undergoing either laproscopic cholecystectomy, open cholecystectomy, or general anesthesia without surgery (controls). They found markedly elevated serum levels of ACTH immediately after surgery in the animals who had received laparoscopic surgery compared to those who received open surgery and controls. There was a significant difference ($p < 0.05$) when the laparoscopic group was compared to the control group. The difference was less significant ($p < 0.02$) when the laparoscopic group was compared to the open group. Cortisol was significantly elevated in the laparoscopic group when compared to both the open group ($p < 0.03$) and the control group ($p < 0.005$). Serum insulin and glucagon varied widely and no significant differences were seen between groups. The authors conclude that laparoscopy is at least as stressful, if not more so, than laparotomy. These results confirm the results of Cooper et al. who found significant elevations of stress-related hormones (cortisol, prolactin, growth hormone and serum glucose levels) on completion of laparoscopy in 22 healthy women [39]. Mansour et al. postulate that the creation and maintenance of the pneumoperitoneum may be responsible for the hormonal differences as, other than the skin incisions, no portion of the laparoscopic operation differed from the open procedure. Both groups hypothesized that acute stretch of the peritoneum by carbon dioxide insufflation may activate receptors which trigger ACTH and cortisol release. It has also been proposed that vasovagal reactions may occur with insufflation and peritoneal stretching, causing a neural stimulus for hormonal release. This is clinically supported by observations of cardiac arrhythmias, including bradycardia and sinus arrest, with peritoneal insufflation [42–44].

The stress response to open versus laparoscopic cholecystectomy was subsequently studied by Milheiro et al. [45] in humans in a prospective randomized study of 40 patients. Both serum cortisol and renin levels were measured. Blood samples were taken prior to and during surgery, as well as on postoperative days 1 and 2. A significant rise in cortisol and renin levels was seen during and after laparoscopic and open surgery with no statistically significant difference between the two surgical approaches. Again, despite the clinical observation that patients recover from laparoscopy with a more comfortable and more rapid postoperative course, laparoscopy appears not to lessen the hormonal stress response as measured by the parameters used in this study.

The human stress response accompanying laparoscopic cholecystectomy compared to open cholecystectomy was further elucidated by Deuss et al. [21], who measured perioperative and intra-operative levels of ACTH, cortisol, prolactin, and growth hormone. ACTH levels became maximally elevated after skin incision and cortisol levels became maximally elevated 2 h after extubation. The maximum ACTH and cortisol levels were greater for the laparoscopic group; however, these differences were not statistically significant. The authors propose that peritoneal incision is the major stimulus for ACTH and cortisol secretion, independent of the size of the skin incision. However, the basis for this conclusion is not obvious. Blood levels were not obtained after establishment of pneumoperitoneum and before skin closure in the laparoscopic group. Therefore, no statement could be made with regard to the possible contribution of the iatrogenic pneumoperitoneum to the rise in ACTH and cortisol levels.

The response pattern of serum prolactin levels was similar in both the open and laparoscopic groups. Intubation resulted in significant increase in prolactin, which is consistent with existing data on general anesthesia and prolactin secretion. Maximum prolactin levels were observed directly after peritoneal incision in the laparoscopic group and 30 min after extubation in the open group. Levels returned to normal as early as 5 h after extubation in both groups.

Serum growth hormone levels reached maximum levels after skin closure in the laparoscopic group. The growth hormone response was very nonhomogenous in the open group. Analysis of growth hormone in the open group was further confounded as four patients had markedly elevated levels preoperatively.

Deuss et al. [21] conclude that laparoscopic cholecystectomy is associated with a significant endocrine stress response which is comparable to that observed in patients undergoing conventional cholecystectomy. Analysis of the results of this study is limited by its non-randomized study design and two groups of patients which are not truly comparable. Only 12 of 65 patients underwent conventional cholecystectomy. The patients in the conventional group generally had more severe biliary disease and three of the 12 had to be converted from a laparoscopic procedure to the open surgical approach.

Targarona et al. recently compared the neuroendocrine and acute phase responses after laparoscopic versus open cholecystectomy [46]. A total of 12 patients underwent laparoscopic cholecystectomy and 13 patients underwent open cholecystectomy. All patients had uncomplicated cholelithiasis. All patients were considered low surgical risk (ASA I or II, American Society of Anesthesiogists). Serum ACTH, cortisol, growth hormone, glucagon, and insulin levels were measured. Cholecystectomy performed by either approach was accompanied by a significant increase in all hormonal levels measured (times not specified). The rise in ACTH and cortisol was greater in the open group; however, this difference was not significant. Once again, this study confirms that cholecystectomy performed by open or laparoscopic surgery induces a significant injury response which is equivalent regardless of technique.

O'Leary et al. performed a study in 16 consecutive patients undergoing laparoscopic cholecystectomy to specifically examine the effect of the pneumoperitoneum on the neuroendocrine response [47]. Plasma levels of prolactin, growth hormone, epinephrine, norepinephrine, cortisol, and renin-aldosterone were measured before and after induction of anesthesia, before and after insufflation, after reverse-Trendelenberg positioning, and after exsufflation. The authors demonstrated a maximal increase in prolactin after induction of general anesthesia. Cortisol, epinephrine, and growth hormone increased with pneumoperitoneum, but was maximal and most significant after exsufflation. The authors conclude that the maximal stimulus to epinephrine, cortisol, and growth hormone secretion is not pneumoperitoneum, but rather the drugs used for reversal of anesthesia, return to consciousness, and postoperative pain and anxiety (i.e., postoperative stress).

In contrast, the increase in renin and aldosterone plasma concentrations were clearly and temporally related to abdominal insufflation and pneumoperitoneum. The authors propose that pneumoperitoneum causes reduced venous return, compression of abdominal capacitance vessels, reduced cardiac output, and decreased renal blood flow leading to activation of the renin-aldosterone system. This hypothesis is similar to that proposed by Le Roith et al. when they demonstrated increased ADH levels with experimental models of increased intra-abdominal pressure [30]. This study once again sheds doubt on the presumption that laparoscopy minimizes the neurohormonal response to surgery.

The hypothesis that laparoscopy produces an attenuated hormonal stress response compared to the open surgical approach was finally tested in a prospective and randomized fashion by Ortega et al. [48]. A total of 20 otherwise healthy women, between ages 18 and 45, with a history of uncomplicated cholelithiasis underwent either laparoscopic ($n = 10$) or open ($n = 10$) cholecystectomy. The classical hormonal stress response was measured, including the adrenocortical (serum ACTH, cortisol, urinary free cortisol), adrenomedullary (plasma and urinary epinephrine and norepinephrine), and pituitary (ADH and growth hormone) hormonal axis, as well as the components of glucose metabolism (serum glucose, glucagon, and insulin). Measurements were made serially (ten measurements) over a 24-h period.

Serum ADH levels were highest intraoperatively during insufflation, and were significantly higher in the laparoscopic group ($p < 0.01$). The authors support the previously proposed hypotheses that the mechanism may lie with stretch or pressure receptors in the peritoneum [31], or alternatively, with decreased venous return and stimulation of intrathoracic volume receptors [28, 30, 32]. Growth hormone levels were similar in the two groups.

Serum ACTH levels rose intraoperatively and peaked during the first 4 postoperative hours in both groups; however, the postoperative deviation from baseline tended to be higher in the open group. Cortisol levels were slightly elevated in the immediate postoperative period with both groups having a similar response pattern.

Plasma epinephrine and norepinephrine levels were very similar between the two groups; however, they tended to be higher intraoperatively and immediately postoperatively in the laparoscopic group. These findings are consistent with those of Mealy et al. [41], who found higher urinary vanilmandelic acid (VMA) levels in the patients undergoing laparoscopic cholecystectomy and suggest that laparoscopy may result in increased catabolic hormone release. On the other hand, one may compare the results of Ortega et al. to those of Joris et al. who also found no significant difference in cortisol or catecholamine concentrations between laparoscopic and open cholecystectomy patients [49].

Intraoperative glucose levels were greater in the laparoscopic group, while postoperative glucose and insulin levels were greater in the open group. If one considers glucose metabolism as the final pathway of the neuroendocrine response to injury, these results, as well as the adrenocortical data, may then suggest that laparoscopic cholecystectomy is more stressful intraoperatively, and less stressful postoperatively when compared to the open technique.

Once again, the hypothesis that the laparoscopic technique is a less "stressful" approach to surgical problems is not fully substantiated by the analysis of the hormonal responses presented in this small, but well designed, study.

Neuroendocrine studies which use cholecystectomy as the model surgical procedure have been criticized as inadequate in design to properly compare the stress response between open and laparoscopic surgery. Mack criticizes the use of the cholecystectomy model when documenting the neuroendocrine and metabolic stress responses to surgery [50], stating that cholecystectomy is a relatively minor procedure which does not create a significantly negative nitrogen balance [41] and is, therefore, not adequate to study the hormonal or metabolic response to laparoscopic versus open surgical procedures. Milheiro responds with the suggestion that similar studies be performed with other laparoscopic procedures such as colon or gastric surgery [51]. However, Delgado et al. [52], Harmon et al. [53], and Bessler et al. [54] have demonstrated that the adrenocortical response to laparoscopic colectomy ,as measured by serum cortisol levels, is not significantly different between the laparoscopic and open surgical approaches.

Conclusions

Laparoscopy is associated with a significant hormonal stress response. This response involves the classical stress hormones elucidated by the hypothalamic-pituitary-adrenal axis as well as the regulatory components of glucose metabolism. Controversy abounds when attempts are made to compare the injury response of laparoscopy to that of conventional surgery. Attempts to confirm the postulate that laparoscopy results in an attenuated surgical neuroendocrine stress response have generally not been successful. Most of the available data suggest that there is no significant hormonal difference between the two surgical approaches, despite the presumption that laparoscopy causes less direct tissue injury. It is perhaps symbolic and fitting that the term "minimally invasive surgery" has given way to the more accurate designation of "minimal access surgery." Conventional surgery usually involves a larger skin incision, greater muscular destruction, increased third-space losses due to an exposed abdominal cavity, greater manipulation of the bowel, and is accompanied by more postoperative pain. Laparoscopy involves an iatrogenic pneumoperitoneum, increased

Table 2.   Stress-related factors during cholecystectomy

Operative parameter	Laparoscopic	Open
Length of operation	↑	↓
Length of incision	↓	↑
Position	↑[a]	↓[b]
Visceral Retraction	↓	↑
Tissue dessication	↓	↑
Tissue destruction	↓	↑
Pneumoperitoneum	+	-
Peritoneal stretch	↑	↓
Intra-abdominal pressure	↑	↓
CO_2/acidosis	+	-
Hemodynamic/ Respiratory compromise	↑	↓

↑ Increased; ↓ decreased; + present; - absent
[a] Reverse-Trendelenberg
[b] Supine

abdominal pressure, altered acid-base balance due to carbon dioxide insuffla-tion, and altered circulatory and pulmonary mechanics. The contribution of any single parameter (such as pneumoperitoneum) to the neurohormonal response is inherently difficult to define and measure (see Table 2).

The complexity of the resultant neurohormonal response becomes increas-ingly evident as one attempts to analyze the data generated by the various ani-mal and human studies currently existing in the literature. It is clear, however, that any differences in the neurohormonal stress response between laparoscopy and conventional surgery which do exist are subtle. This leads one to question how clinically relevant is the difference in the magnitude or pattern of neuroen-docrine response. Clearly, the improved postoperative course of the laparoscopic patient in terms of discomfort and overall morbidity can not be explained by differences in the response of the reviewed endocrine parameters. This leads one to question whether more relevant biochemical parameters should be sought. There is, in fact, an increasing body of data which suggest that the acute-phase response – as measured by C-reactive protein (CRP), interleukin-6, and total T lymphocyte count – is attenuated after laparoscopic surgical procedures [40, 46]. It is perhaps those studies which demonstrate an attenuated acute phase response after laparoscopic cholecystectomy which best support the concept that the laparoscopic procedure is less traumatic. Data concerning the neurohormonal and acute phase responses to laparoscopy are only now becoming readily avail-able. Continued investigation into the neurologic, hormonal, acute phase, and immune responses to laparoscopy may provide a scientific foundation for the improved clinical outcome observed after laparoscopic surgery.

References

1. McMahon AJ, Russell IT, Baxter JN, Ross S, Anderson JR, Morran CG, Sunderland G, Galloway D, Ramsay G, O'Dwyer PJ (1994) Laparoscopic versus minilaparotomy cholecystectomy: a randomized trial. Lancet 343:135–138
2. Attwood SE, Hill AD, Mealy K, Stephens RB (1992) A prospective comparison of laparoscopic versus open cholecystectomy. Ann R Coll Surg Engl 74:397–400
3. Burch JM, Moore EE, Moore FA, Francoise R (1996) The abdominal compartment syndrome. Surg Clin North Am 76:833–842
4. Schein M, Wittman DH, Aprahamian CC, Condon RE (1995) The abdominal compartment syndrome: the physiological and clinical consequences of elevated intra-abdominal pressure. J Am Coll Surg 180:745–753
5. Hunter JG (1995) Laparoscopic pneumoperitoneum: the abdominal compartment syndrome revisited. J Am Coll Surg 181:469–470
6. Bendahan J, Coetzee C, Papagianopoulos C, Muller R (1995) Abdominal compartment syndrome. J Trauma 381:152–153
7. Eddy VA, Key SP, Morris JA (1994) Abdominal compartment syndrome: etiology, detection and management. J Tenn Med Assoc 87:55–57
8. Safran DB, Orlando R (1994) Physiologic effects of pneumoperitoneum. Am J Surg 167:281–286
9. Callery MP, Soper NJ (1993) Physiology of the pneumoperitoneum. In: Bailliere T (ed) Bailliere's clinical gastroenterology, vol 7/4. Bailliere Tindall, London, pp 757–777
10. Scott-Conner CEH, Hardy JD (1988) Response to surgery: neuroendocrine and metabolic changes, convalescence, and rehabilitation. In: Hardy JD (ed) Hardy's textbook of surgery, 2nd edn. Lippincott, Philadelphia, pp 3–13
11. Kehlet H (1978) Influences of epidural analgesia on the endocrine-metabolic response to surgery. Acta Aneaesth Scan Suppl 70:39–42
12. Hagen C, Brandt MR, Kehlet H (1980) Prolactin, LH, FSH, and cortisol response to surgery and the effect of epidural analgesia. Acta Endocrinol 94:151–154
13. Engquist A, Brandt MR, Fernandes A, Kehlet H (1977) The blocking effect of epidural analgesia on the adrenocortical and hyperglycemic responses to surgery. Acta Aneaesth Scan 21:330–335
14. Brandt M, Kehlet H, Binder C, Hagen C, McNeilly AS (1976) Effect of epidural analgesia on the glycoregulatory and endocrine response to surgery. Clin Endocrinol 5:107–114
15. Verney EB (1947) The antidiuretic hormone and the factors which determine its release. Proc R Soc Lond 135:25–106
16. Orr J, Snaith AH (1959) A method for the estimation of antidiuretic hormone in urine. J Endocrinol 18:16
17. Moran WH, Miltenberger FW (1963) Use of the intravenous route for maintenance of water balance in the alcoholized rat bioassay of vasopressin. Fed Proc 22:386
18. Moran WH, Zimmerman B (1967) Mechanisms of antidiuretic hormone (ADH) control of importance to the surgical patient. Surgery 62:639–644
19. Moran WH, Miltenberger FW, Shuaye WA, Zimmerman B (1964) The relationship of antidiuretic hormone secretion to surgical stress. Surgery 56:99–108
20. Cochrane JPS, Forsling ML, Menzies Gow N, Le Quesne LP (1981) Arginine vassopressin release following surgical operations. Br J Surg 68:209–213
21. Deusss U, Dietrich J, Kaulen D, Frey K, Spangenberger W, Allolio B, Matuszczak M, Troidl H, Winkelmann W (1994) The stress response to laparoscopic cholecystectomy: investigation of endocrine parameters. Endoscopy 26:235–238
22. Noel GL, Suh HK, Stone G, Frants AG (1972) Human prolactin and growth hormone release during surgery and other conditions of stress. J Clin Endocrinol Metab 35:84–851
23. Sowers JR, Raj RP, Hershman JM, Carlson HE, McCallum RW (1977) The effect of stressful diagnostic studies and surgery on the anterior pituitary hormone release in man. Acta Endocrinol 86:25–32
24. Targarona M, Balague C, Espert JJ, Caceres JP, Gaya J et al (1994) Laparoscopic cholecystectomy induces an attenuated metabolic response to surgical injury. A comparative study with open cholecystectomy. SAGES abstract: 111

25. Mansour MA, Stiegmann GV, Yamamoto M, Berguer R (1992) Neuroendocrine stress response after minimally invasive surgery in pigs. Surg Endosc 6:294–297
26. Cryer PE (1980) Physiology and pathophysiology of the human sympathoadrenal neuroendocrine system. N Engl J Med 303:436–444
27. Allson AP, Tomlin PJ (1969) Some effects of aneaesthesia and surgery on carbohydrate and fat metabolism. Br J Anaesth 42:588–93
28. Husain MK, Manger WM, Rock TW, Weiss RJ, Frantz AG (1979) Vasopressin release due to manual restrain in the rat: role of body compression and comparison with other stressful stimuli. Endocrinology 10:641–644
29. Forsling ML, Ullman E (1974) Release of vasopressin during hypoxia. J Phsiol 241:35P-36P
30. Le Roith D, Bark M, Glick SM (1982) The effect of abdominal pressure on plasma antidiuretic hormone levels in the dog. J Surg Res 32:65–69
31. Punnonen R, Viinamaki O (1982) Vasopressin release during laparoscopy: role of increased intra-abdominal pressure. Lancet 1:175–176
32. Melville RJ, Frizis HI, Forsling ML, LeQuesne LP (1985) The stimulus for vasopressin release during laparoscopy. Surg Obstet Gynecol 161:253–256
33. Herruzo JA, Castellano G, Larrodera L, Morillas JD, Sanchez DM, Provencio R, Munoz-Yague MT (1989) Plasma arginine vasopressin concentration during laparoscopy. Hepatogastroenterology 36:499–503
34. Schultz HD, Fater DC, Sundet WD, Geer PG, Goetz KL (1982) Reflexes elicited by acute stretch of atrial vs pulmonary receptors in conscious dogs. Am J Physiol 242:H1065-H1076
35. Voltz J, Koster S, Weiss M, Schmidt R, Urbaschek R, Melchert F, Albrecht M (1996) Pathophysiologic features of a pneumoperitoneum at laparoscopy: a swine model. Am J Obstet Gynecol 174:132–140
36. Bonnet F, Harari A, Thibonnier M (1982) Vasopressin response to pneumoperitoneum: mechanical of nociceptive stimulation. Lancet 1:452
37. Hunter JG (1995) Laparoscopic pneumoperitoneum: The abdominal compartment syndrome revisited. J Am Coll Surg 181:469–470
38. Rutkow JM (1987) Surgical operations in the United States: 1979–1984. Surgery 101:192–200
39. Cooper GM , Scoggins AM, Ward ID, Murphy D (1982) Laparoscopy – a stressful procedure. Anaesth 37:266–269
40. Dionigi R, Dominioni L, Benevento A, Giudice G, Cuffari S, Bordone N, Caravati F, Carcano G, Gennari R (1994) Effects of surgical trauma of laparoscopic vs open cholecystectomy. Hepatogastroenterology 41:471–476
41. Mealy K, Gallagher H, Barry M, Lennon F, Traynor O, Hyland J (1992) Physiological and metabolic responses to open and laparoscopic cholecystectomy. Br J Surg 79:1061-1064
42. Shifren JL, Adlestein L, Finkler NJ (1992) Asystolic cardiac arrest: a rare complication of laparoscopy. Obstet Gynecol 79:840–841
43. Doyle DJ, Mark PWS (1990) Reflex bradycardia during surgery. Can J Anaesth 37:219–22
44. Carmichael DE (1971) Laparoscopy-cardiac considerations. Fertil Steril 22:69–70
45. Milheiro A, Sousa FC, Manso EC, Leitao F (1994) Metabolic responses to cholecystectomy: open vs laparoscopic approach. J Laparoendosc Surg 4:311–317
46. Targarona EM, Pons MJ, Balague C, Esper JJ, Moral A, Martinez J, Gaya J, Filella X, Rivera F, Ballestra A, Trias M (1996) Acute phase is the only significantly reduced component of the injury response after laparoscopic cholecystectomy. World J Surg 20:528–534
47. O'Leary E, Hubbard K, Tormey W, Cunningham AJ (1996) Laparoscopic cholecystectomy: hemodynamic and neuroendocrine responses after pneumoperitoneum and changes in position. Br J Anaesth 76:640–644
48. Ortega AE, Peters JH, Incarbone R, Estrada L, Ehsan A, Kwan Y, Spencer CJ, Moore-Jeffries E, Kuchta K, Nicoloff JT (1996) A prospective randomized comparison of the metabolic and stress hormonal responses of laparoscopic and open cholecystectomy. J Am Coll Surg 183:249–256
49. Joris J, Ciganrini I, Legrnad M, Jacquet N, De Groote D, Franchimont P, Lamy M (1992) Metabolic and respiratory changes after cholecystectomy performed via laparotomy or laparoscopy. Br J Anaesth 69:341–345
50. Mack P (1994) Metabolic responses to cholecystectomy: open versus laparoscopic. J Laparoendosc Surg 5:207–208

51. Milheiro A (1994) Metabolic responses to cholecystectomy: open versus laparoscopic. J Laparo-endosc Surg 5:208–209
52. Delgado S, Lacy AM, Garcia-Valdecasas JC, Filella A, Anglada T, Grande L, Fuster J, Pique JM, Visa J (1996) Comparison of metabolic responses to laparoscopic and open cholecystectomy in a randomized trial (abstract). Fifth World Congress of Endoscopic Surgery, Philadelphia, 13–17 March 1996
53. Harmon G, Senagore A, Kilbride M, Luchtefeld M, MacKeigan J, Warzynski M (1993) Cortisol and IL-6 response attenuated following laparoscopic colectomy. Surg Endosc (abstract) 7:121
54. Bessler M, Whelan RL, Halverson A, Treat MR, Nowygrod R (1994) Is immune function better preserved after laparoscopic versus open colon resection? Surg Endosc 8:881–883

12 Monitoring and Management of Physiological Changes Caused by Pneumoperitoneum

I. Azar

Introduction

The introduction of therapeutic laparoscopic procedures has been associated with several physiological changes and complications that were not encountered in conventional surgery. These include respiratory and hemodynamic embarrassment, hypercarbia, gas embolism, pneumothorax, pulmonary aspiration of gastric contents, cardiac arrhythmias, and increased intracranial pressure (ICP). These changes and complications are primarily caused by increased intra-abdominal pressure during the establishment of pneumoperitoneum (PP) [1–3].

As a general rule, we can say that the lower the insufflation pressure during laparoscopy the lower the incidence of PP complications [4]. The insufflation pressure, therefore, should be kept as low as possible. This is particularly important since little is gained from high insufflation pressure. As the insufflation pressure increases, the gain in abdominal volume per unit of pressure decreases [5]. Higher insufflation pressures do not facilitate the insertion of trocar or needles through the abdominal wall. Based on these findings, the recommended maximal insufflation pressure is 15 mmHg.

The overall incidence of serious complications during laparoscopic surgery is low [3]. It can be further reduced by continually monitoring respiratory and cardiovascular functions during peritoneal insufflation. Early detection and prompt preventive and therapeutic measures may contain the complications and improve patient outcome.

The purpose of this chapter is to review monitoring techniques,as well as preventive measures and treatment for PP complications during laparoscopy.

Ventilatory Embarrassment

PP may embarrass ventilation by two mechanisms:
1. The increased intra-abdominal pressure interferes with the free movement of the diaphragm [6] and thus reduces ventilation at the base of the lungs [7]. Since most of the pulmonary gas exchange occurs at the base of the lungs, this may have an adverse effect on blood oxygenation. Although there have been no reports of hypoxemia during laparoscopy, it is conceivable that this complication may occur in patients with marginal pulmonary function.

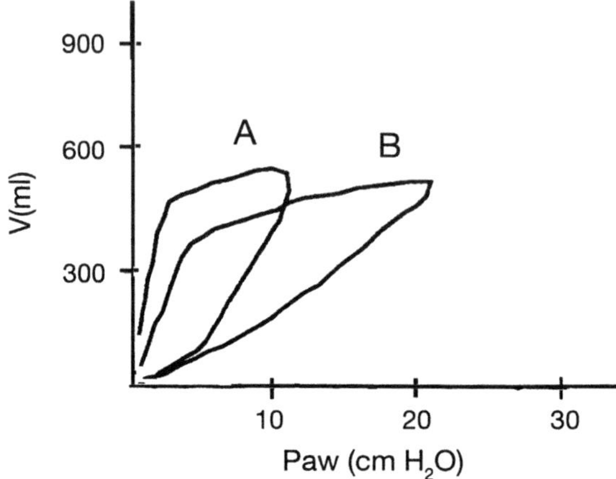

Fig. 1. Changes in total respiratory compliance during pneumoperitoneum for laparoscopic cholecystectomy. (The intra-abdominal pressure was 14 mmHg and the head-up tilt 10°). Illustration of the airway pressure (Paw) versus volume (V) curves and data were obtained from the screeen of a Datex Ultima before insufflation (*A*) and 30 min after insufflation (*B*). (From [71])

2. The increased intra-abdominal pressure decreases chest compliance and thus increases peak airway pressure (Fig. 1). As a result, the bronchial tree may expand during positive pressure ventilation and increase the pulmonary physiological dead space. If indeed the dead space increases, the tidal volume must be increased to avoid hypercarbia. Some authors have found an increase in dead space during laparoscopy [7, 8], while others have not [9].

An increase in airway pressure during laparoscopy may pose additional dangers to patients with chronic obstructive pulmonary disease. These patients often have hyperactive airway and lung bullae. During laparoscopy, the airway pressure may be particularly high in these patients, leading to an excessive fall in cardiac output (see below) and pneumothorax may occur due to rupture of lung bullae.

Monitoring Ventilatory Effects

The effects of PP on ventilation can be monitored as follows (Fig. 2):
1. The pressure gauge of the anesthesia breathing circuit indicates circuit pressure during the breathing cycle. This pressure correlates with peak airway pressure. When chest compliance is normal the peak breathing circuit pressure is 5–15 cm/H_2O. A rise in the peak pressure to above 20 cm/H_2O suggests either airway obstruction, mechanical problems in the breathing circuit, or poor chest compliance. During laparoscopy a rise in airway pressure may be due to an increase in intra-abdominal pressure and a decrease in chest compliance.
2. Pulse oximetry is a noninvasive and easy method of beat-to-beat monitoring of hemoglobin O_2 saturation. The device continually displays the heart rate and O_2 saturation. A fall in O_2 saturation during laparoscopy suggests reduced ventilation at the base of the lungs and increased ventilation/perfusion mismatch due to PP interference with diaphragmatic excursion.

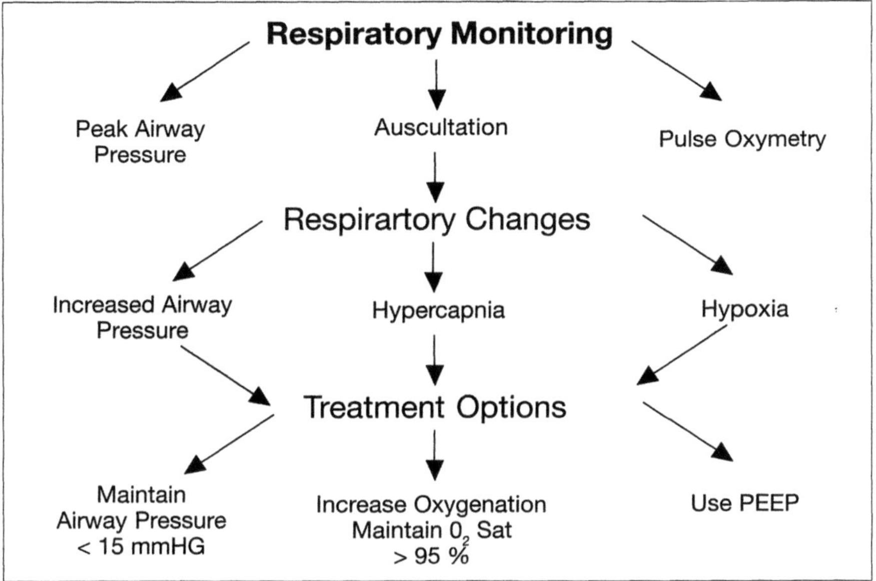

Fig. 2. Algorithm for respiratory monitoring during laparoscopic procedures. PEEP, positive end-expiratory pressure; Sat, saturation

Prevention and Treatment of Ventilatory Effects

Although PP increases airway pressure and may decrease O_2 saturation, other causes of hypoxemia should be considered when it occurs during laparoscopy. Breath sounds should be checked to rule out inadvertent endobronchial intubation, bronchospasm, pulmonary atelectasis, or pneumothorax. In addition, inadequate inspiratory O_2 concentration, breathing circuit malfunction, and gas embolism should be ruled out (see below).

If ventilatory embarrassment and hypoxemia occur during laparoscopy, the following corrective measures are recommended:

1. Maintain the insufflation pressure at or below 15 mmHg.
2. Gradually increase the inspiratory O_2 concentration until the hemoglobin O_2 saturation rises above 95%.
3. Apply positive end-expiratory pressure (PEEP) to the breathing circuit. This will open collapsed alveoli at the base of the lungs and improve blood oxygenation. However, if the patient's airway pressure is already excessive, PEEP may reduce the cardiac output and increase the risk of pneumothorax.

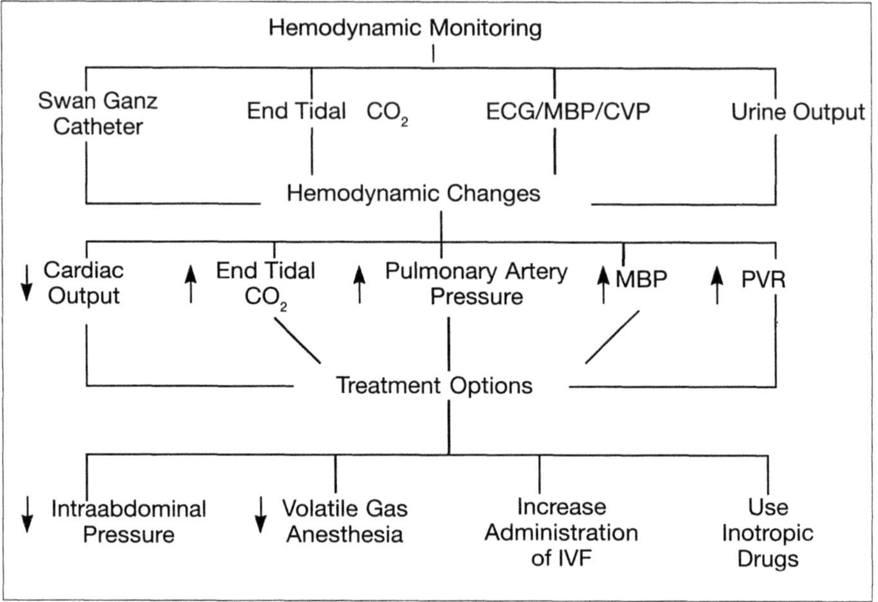

Fig. 3. Algorithm for hemodynamic monitoring during laparoscopic procedures. ECG, electrocardiography; MBP, mean blood pressure; CVP, central venous pressure; PVR, pulmonary venous pressure; IVF, intravascular fluid

Hemodynamic Embarrassment

Hemodynamic embarrassment occurs during laparoscopic surgery when the intra-abdominal pressure rises above 10 mmHg (Fig. 3) [10–13]. Characteristically, the cardiac output decreases and systemic vascular resistance (SVR) and pulmonary resistance, as well as arterial blood pressure, increase (Fig. 4). A combination of general anesthesia, an insufflation pressure of 14 mmHg, and head-down position can reduce the cardiac output by 50% [10]. The fall in cardiac output is proportional to the intra-abdominal pressure and is seen in all patients regardless of their position on the operating table [11].

The cause of the fall in cardiac output during laparoscopy is multifactorial. One of the more important factors is a reduction in inferior vena cava blood flow caused by pooling of blood in the legs [11, 14, 15]. The decline in cardiac output parallels the reduction in venous return [11]. However, despite the fall in venous return, the cardiac filling pressures increase [10, 16, 17]. This is due to a concomitant increase in intrathoracic pressure. The net result is a decrease in right atrial transmural pressure and, therefore, a fall in cardiac output [10, 16, 18].

The increase in SVR during laparoscopy is primarily a reaction to the fall in cardiac output; however, the increase persists after the abdomen has been de-

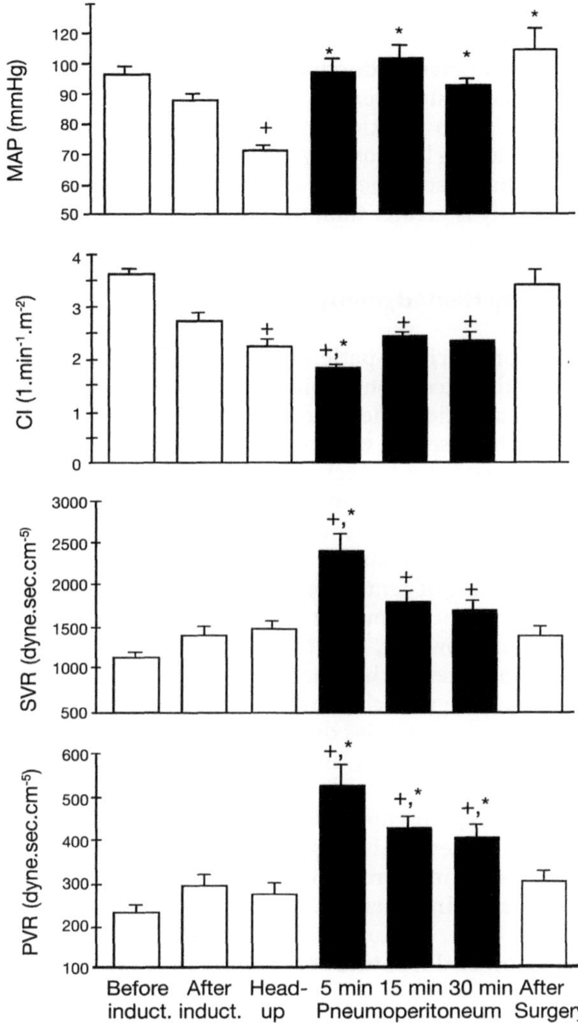

Fig. 4. Hemodynamic changes during laparoscopic cholecystectomy. MAP, mean arterial pressure; CI, cardiac index; SVR, systemic vascular resistance; PVR, pulmonary venous pressure

flated and the cardiac output returned to baseline [19]. There has been speculation that the compression of abdominal vessels triggers the release of humoral factors such as catecholamines, prostaglandins, renin, and vasopressin [20, 21]. These substances linger in the body for some time after decompression of the abdomen and maintain elevated SVR postoperatively.

The increase in intra-abdominal pressure during laparoscopy also affects renal function. In one study, when the abdominal pressure was raised to 20 mmHg, the renal vascular resistance increased by 500% and the glomerular filtration rate decreased by more than 75% [22, 23]. Even insufflation pressure as low as 15 mmHg can reduce cortical renal blood flow by 60% and cause oliguria. However, no permanent reduction in renal function has been reported even in patients with end-stage renal disease.

In addition to the kidneys, the blood supply of all other abdominal organs decreases during laparoscopy, with the exception of the adrenal glands [24]. This includes the mesenteric and intestinal blood flow. The fall in abdominal organ blood supply is greater than the fall in cardiac output, suggesting regional vasoconstriction.

Monitoring Hemodynamic Effects

In the vast majority of patients, the hemodynamic effects of PP are inconsequential. With the exception of blood pressure and electrocardiogram (ECG) monitoring, most patients need no hemodynamic monitoring. The renal effects of PP can easily be assessed by monitoring urinary output. Roughly 1 ml/kg per hour of urinary output is expected during surgery.

There are no reports in the literature on the hemodynamic effects of PP in patients with cardiac disorders. Indirect evidence suggests these patients sustain greater hemodynamic changes than usual [7]. It is recommended, therefore, that monitoring of central venous (CVP) and pulmonary artery (PAP) pressures, as well as cardiac output, be considered for patients with severely compromised circulation. However, due to the increase in intra-thoracic pressure during laparoscopy, interpreting changes in CVP and PAP may be difficult.

Transesophageal echocardiography might be particularly useful in cardiac patients since it provides direct information on filling volumes of the heart and myocardial contractility, and it can detect gas emboli in the central circulation.

End-tidal CO_2 monitoring is also useful in the assessment of cardiac function during laparoscopy. A fall in cardiac output is often associated with a fall in end-tidal CO_2 level. Although CO_2 absorption from the peritoneal cavity might complicate the interpretation of end-tidal CO_2 level changes, the trend may still provide useful information.

Prevention and Treatment of Hemodynamic Effects

Hemodynamic embarrassment during laparoscopy can be minimized by reducing the insufflation pressure. This is particularly important in patients with cardiac disorders or hypovolemia. If PP causes an excessive fall in cardiac output and blood pressure the insufflation pressure, firstly, should be reduced to the lowest possible level. Secondly, since volatile inhalation anesthesia depresses myocardial contractility, it should be discontinued and intravenous anesthesia used instead. If the blood pressure remains low, an intravenous fluid challenge should be tried. Finally, a bolus of an inotropic agent followed by continuous infusion of the medication might be necessary to boost the circulation.

If there are signs of decreased renal function, intravenous hydration should first be tried. If this does not improve the urinary output, a dopamine drip in "renal" doses is recommended [25].

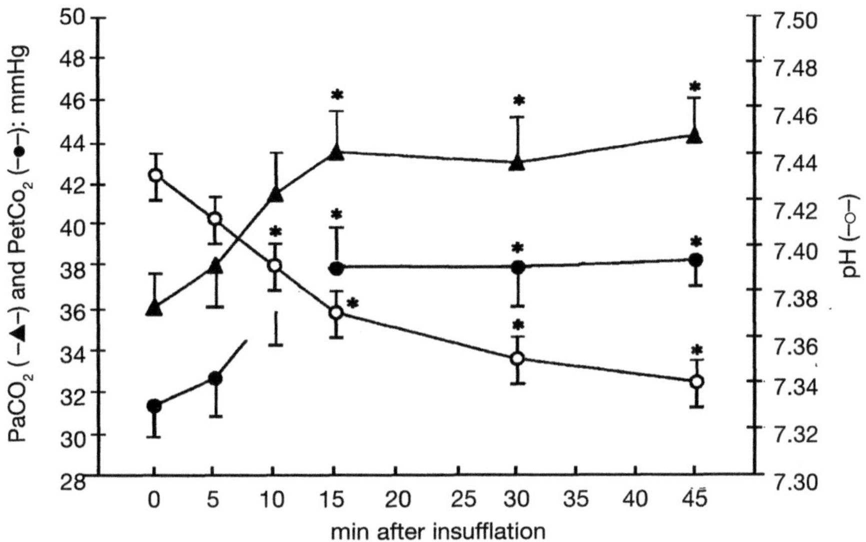

Fig. 5. Ventilatory changes (pH, $PaCO_2$, $PETCO_2$) during CO_2 pneumoperitoneum for laparoscopic cholecystectomy Intra-abdominal pressure was 14 mmHg. Data are mean ± SEM. *$p < .05$ as compared with time 0. (From [72])

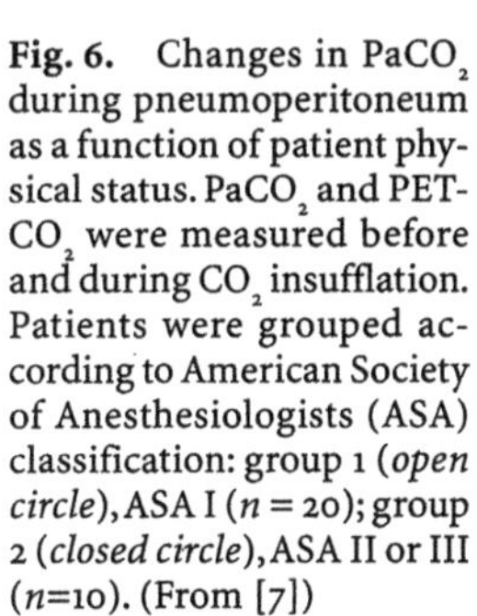

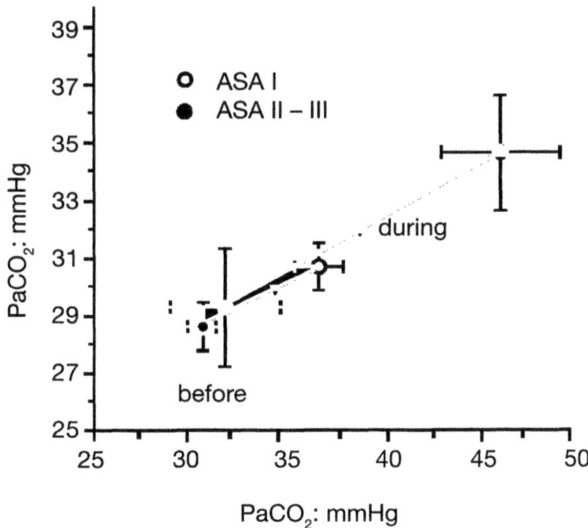

Fig. 6. Changes in $PaCO_2$ during pneumoperitoneum as a function of patient physical status. $PaCO_2$ and $PETCO_2$ were measured before and during CO_2 insufflation. Patients were grouped according to American Society of Anesthesiologists (ASA) classification: group 1 (*open circle*), ASA I ($n = 20$); group 2 (*closed circle*), ASA II or III ($n=10$). (From [7])

Hypercarbia

CO_2 is the most commonly used gas for abdominal insufflation during laparoscopy. It is a highly soluble gas and rapidly diffuses from the peritoneal cavity into the preperitoneal blood vessels. As a result, when the patient is under general anesthesia and receiving constant ventilation, a rise in arterial PCO_2 usually occurs (Fig. 5).

The incidence of hypercarbia during laparoscopy depends on the insufflation pressure and on the duration of the procedure [16]. The higher the pressure, the greater the incidence and level of hypercarbia. If surgery is brief, the hypercarbia is usually insignificant; however, if it is prolonged, a significant rise in arterial PCO_2 may occur.

Patients with cardiopulmonary disorders sustain a greater than usual rise in arterial PCO_2 during laparoscopy [7] (Fig. 6). The rate of peritoneal CO_2 absorption during laparoscopy is limited due to a reduction in cardiac output (see above). As the intra-abdominal pressure increases at the beginning of the procedure, the cardiac output falls and the rate of peritoneal CO_2 absorption decreases. At the conclusion of the procedure, as the abdomen is being deflated, there is usually a surge in cardiac output. As a result, peritoneal CO_2 absorption increases [26] and CO_2 mobilization from body stores occurs [27]. This transiently increases the end-tidal CO_2 level.

Another possible contributory factor to the hypercarbia observed during laparoscopy is the ventilatory impairment caused by the patient's position [8, 28]. Steep Trendelenburg positioning further decreases chest compliance as the abdominal contents push against the diaphragm compressing the lower lobes of the lungs and decreasing the ventilation perfusion ratio. The latter will further increase hypercarbia.

Monitoring CO_2 Blood Level

The most common and practical method for monitoring the blood CO_2 level during laparoscopy is the breath-to-breath capnography. The end-tidal CO_2 level approximately represents the arterial PCO_2. However, because of physiological shunting in the lungs, the end-tidal CO_2 level is always lower than the arterial PCO_2. The greater the ventilation-perfusion mismatch, the greater the discrepancy between the two parameters. In most patients, this difference is no greater than 10 mmHg.

End-tidal CO_2 monitoring during general anesthesia has become standard care in the operating room. The New York State Health Code mandates it. There are several different technologies for end-tidal CO_2 analysis, but the simplest and most commonly used one is based on infrared analysis. Modern operating rooms are equipped with capnograms that continuously draw samples of respiratory gases from the anesthesia breathing circuit and determine the end-tidal CO_2 level.

Prevention and Treatment

In general, hypercarbia is far less hazardous than hypoxemia. Patients are able to tolerate a 20% increase in arterial partial pressure of CO_2 with no ill effects.

Only patients with increased intracranial pressure or irritable myocardium and ectopic beats have low tolerance to elevated arterial PCO_2. Since PP tends to increase intracranial pressure (see below), particular care should be taken to maintain a normal arterial PCO_2 in these patients.

In most patients, the increase in PCO_2 during laparoscopy is small and requires no particular therapeutic measures. If necessary, a 10%–25% increase in minute ventilation would easily correct the rise in arterial PCO_2. A greater increase in minute ventilation might be needed if the patient has sustained subcutaneous emphysema, since additional amounts of CO_2 would be absorbed from subcutaneous tissues into the blood stream.

If it is necessary to increase the minute ventilation to maintain a normal CO_2 level during laparoscopy, it is preferable to increase the respiratory rate rather than the tidal volume. This is because an increase in tidal volume will further increase the peak airway pressure. Excessive increase in airway pressure might be particularly problematic in patients with chronic obstructive pulmonary disease (COPD) and bullous emphysema.

Pneumothorax

Increased intraperitoneal pressure during laparoscopy can open embryonic channels to the mediastinum, pleural cavity, and pericardium [29]. This can lead to one- or two-sided pneumothorax, pneumomediastinum, and pneumopericardium, respectively. Often, this is accompanied by subcutaneous emphysema. Defects in the diaphragm around the aortic or esophageal hiatus may also allow gas to diffuse to the mediastinum and from there to the cervical and facial subcutaneous area.

The danger of pneumothorax during laparoscopy in patients with COPD is particularly high since the increase in airway pressure that usually accompanies laparoscopy may cause pre-existing pulmonary bullae to rupture [10, 11].

Detection

The following signs during laparoscopy would suggest peritoneal gas entry into the thoracic cavity:

1. *Excessive progressive rise in airway pressure.* Usually, during laparoscopy, the airway pressure rises moderately and remains stable during surgery. If the pressure continues to rise and this is accompanied by a decrease in O_2 saturation, the possibility of pneumothorax should be considered. The chest should be examined for loss of breath sounds and signs of mediastinal shift.
2. *Rapid decline in blood pressure.* If during laparoscopy the blood pressure falls precipitously and this is accompanied by muffled heart sounds, pneumopericardium should be considered.
3. *Failure of a diaphragmatic leaf to move.* If the surgeon-laparoscopist observes that one of the diaphragmatic leaves is not moving during respiration, this would suggest unilateral pneumothorax during respiration.

Treatment

Tension pneumothorax and/or pneumopericardium may lead to severe cardiopulmonary embarrassment and become life-threatening [30]. If the vital signs start to deteriorate, the insufflation of gas should immediately be discontinued and the abdomen decompressed. If this does not improve the vital signs, a chest tube should be inserted in one or both sides of the chest if necessary. If chest X-rays show pneumopericardium, tapping of the pericardial sac might be necessary.

If a chest tube is inserted laparoscopic surgery must be discontinued since the insufflation gas would otherwise escape through the chest tube. If possible, surgery should be postponed until the patient recovers from the thoracic complications. However, if surgery is urgent or has advanced too far to be abandoned, open conventional surgery should be considered.

If the escape of insufflation gas into the chest cavity causes no cardiopulmonary embarrassment, a chest tube is not necessarily indicated since carbon dioxide is rapidly absorbed [29]. If nitrous oxide is being used for anesthesia, it should be discontinued because of its propensity to diffuse into any collection of gas in the body and expand it. In addition, the discontinuation of nitrous oxide would allow delivery of a higher inspiratory concentration of oxygen. If the patient is still inadequately oxygenated, ventilation should be increased and PEEP added to the breathing circuit before resorting to the insertion of a chest tube.

Gas Embolism

Gas embolism is a rare but often fatal complication of PP [31, 32]. It is more likely to occur when laparoscopy is combined with hysteroscopy [32, 33]. During insufflation, gas may enter the circulation directly if a needle or a trocar accidentally punctures a blood vessel, or indirectly if gas is trapped in the portal circulation [34–39]. Gas embolism can also occur during a surgical procedure [32, 33, 40–43] or postoperatively [44].

Another possible mechanism of gas embolism during laparoscopy is associated with the use of a Nd:YAG laser in conjunction with a gas-cooled sapphire scalpel. During surgery air, CO_2, or nitrogen flow continuously through the scalpel. If the tip of the scalpel accidentally punctures an abdominal blood vessel, gas will flow directly into the circulation [42, 43, 45, 46].

When CO_2 is used for insufflation during laparoscopy, gas embolism rarely occurs since CO_2 easily dissolves or is carried in the blood as carboxyhemoglobin and bicarbonate. The lethal dose of CO_2 is five times greater than that of air [47].

Nevertheless, a large CO_2 embolus can form during laparoscopy and cause a "gas lock" in the vena cava or right atrium [36]. This blocks blood flow from the right side of the heart and abruptly increases right ventricular pressure. The increase in right ventricular pressure may open the foramen ovale, which is patent in 20%–30% of the population [38, 48], and send gas emboli to the brain and coronary circulation [33, 35, 38]. Gas embolism can also increase ventilation-perfusion mismatch and cause hypoxemia by abruptly increasing the physiological dead space of the lungs.

Detection

A sudden rapid decline in vital signs immediately after abdominal insufflation has been started should be considered as a sign of gas embolism until proven otherwise. Signs of accidental penetration of an abdominal vessel with the insufflation needle include blood returning through the hub of the needle, pulsation of CO_2 flowmeter float [35], and failure of the insufflation gas to distend the abdomen [39, 40]. Some investigators [49] have detected bronchospasm, while others [33] have not.

Additional clinical signs of gas embolism include cyanosis, increased breathing circuit pressure, and a sudden rise and then a fall in end-tidal CO_2. The latter is the result of a sudden decrease in pulmonary artery blood flow due to an air lock in the inferior vena cava or right side of the heart [33, 36]. Signs of right heart failure such as distention of neck veins, peripheral cyanosis, and ECG signs of right ventricular strain [50] may also occur. If the embolus is particularly large (2 ml/kg or greater) a wheel murmur may be heard when listening to the heart and cardiac arrhythmias and hypotension may also occur. Pulmonary edema is sometimes an early sign [38, 51].

Advanced monitoring devices such as pulmonary artery line and precordial Doppler can detect signs of gas embolism earlier than conventional monitoring. Doppler monitoring is more sensitive than capnography [39] and both are more sensitive than pulse oximetry. As little as 0.5 ml/kg of gas embolism would change the Doppler sounds and increase the CVP and PAP. However, since gas embolism during laparoscopic procedures is rare and the cost and risks of advanced monitoring significant, the routine use of such monitoring cannot be justified [36, 40, 52].

Prevention and Treatment

Early recognition and treatment of gas embolism improves outcome [35, 47]. The initial flow rate of the insufflation gas should not exceed 1 l/min. If gas embolism is suspected, insufflation should be immediately discontinued, the abdomen deflated, and the patient turned on to the left (right side up) in a steep head-down position. This reduces the amount of gas reaching the right heart [36]. Concomitantly, all inhalation anesthetic agents should be discontinued and O_2 (100%) administered. This will minimize cardiac depression and maximize blood oxygenation [36].

Pulmonary Aspiration

During laparoscopy, the increased intra-abdominal pressure raises the intra-gastric pressure and thus promotes gastric regurgitation. This, in turn, may lead to pulmonary aspiration of gastric contents [53, 54]. Fortunately, the intra-abdominal pressure also increases the competence of the gastro-esophageal sphincter [55, 56], and thus contains the risk of gastric regurgitation. The steep head-down position that is often used during laparoscopic colon procedures further reduces the possibility of pulmonary aspiration.

Despite tracheal intubation with a cuffed tube, seeping of gastric contents around the cuff and pulmonary aspiration is still possible during laparoscopy [57]. The regurgitation of gastric contents may be "silent" and totally missed by the anesthesiologist. Only later, as chemical pneumonitis sets in, would clinical signs of pulmonary aspiration become obvious.

Detection

Typically, following pulmonary aspiration, airway pressure rises and diffuse wheezing may be heard during chest auscultation. Concomitantly, O_2 saturation starts to deteriorate. Suctioning of the pharynx and the endotracheal tube may produce brownish secretions. Arterial blood gas analysis may reveal significant hypoxemia. In contrast, the arterial PCO_2 usually remains normal as long as ventilation is adequate.

Prevention and Treatment

Patients scheduled for laparoscopic surgery are usually premedicated with antacids. Commonly used premedicants include sodium citrate, histamine H_2 blockers, and metoclopromide. After induction of general anesthesia, the airway is secured with a cuffed endotracheal tube. Immediately after intubation, the gastric contents (liquid and gas) is aspirated. This reduces the possibility of regurgitation, as well as accidental perforation of a distended stomach by the surgeon during the insertion of a needle or a trocar through the abdominal wall.

If pulmonary aspiration occurs despite all these precautions, the trachea and the bronchial tree are suctioned thoroughly and, if aspiration of food particles is suspected, fiberoptic bronchoscopy is recommended. Bronchial lavage is not recommended since it has been shown to spread chemical pneumonitis [58].

Postoperatively, the trachea remains intubated and positive pressure ventilation is used until the patient meets extubation criteria. Oxygen supplementation might be necessary to maintain adequate blood oxygenation. Prophylactic antibiotics are also recommended. The use of steroids is controversial and probably useless.

Cardiac Arrhythmias

Although generally associated with acidosis and hypercarbia, cardiac arrhythmias during laparoscopy are more likely to occur when the abdomen is rapidly insufflated at the beginning of the procedure well before the arterial PCO_2 has risen [59]. A possible explanation for these arrhythmias is an increase in vagal tone caused by sudden stretching of the peritoneum in a lightly anesthetized patient [60]. Bradycardia is the most common arrhythmia observed, but ectopic beats and even asystole have also been reported.

Monitoring Cardiac Rhythm

ECG is routinely used during surgery and it is the best monitor of cardiac rhythm. For the purpose of distinguishing between supraventricular and ventricular arrhythmias, lead II is the lead of choice.

Prevention and Treatment

Since halothane is the volatile anesthetic agent most likely to provoke arrhythmia, other volatile agents such as enflurane [61] or isoflurane [62] are preferred for this procedure. To further reduce the incidence of arrhythmias, moderate hyperventilation is recommended in order to maintain a normal CO_2 level.

Although the most likely cause of arrhythmias during laparoscopy is vagal reflex caused by rapid stretching of the peritoneum, other causes should also be considered. Pneumothorax, gas embolism, and hypoxemia should be ruled out (see above). If vagal reflex is suspected, the abdominal insufflation should be discontinued and, if necessary, atropine administered. Once the arrhythmia is corrected, anesthesia can be deepened and the procedure resumed. Some authors advocate prophylactic administration of atropine.

Increased Intracranial Pressure

PP has been shown to raise the ICP in animals [63, 69, 70]. This could be the result of two different mechanisms:
1. Compression of the vena cava by PP raises the central venous pressure and this may reduce cerebral venous return [63, 69].
2. Abdominal insufflation with CO_2 raises the blood CO_2 level and this causes cerebral vasodilatation and increased cerebral blood flow [64, 69].

A transcranial Doppler study of the middle cerebral artery during laparoscopic procedures showed no change in blood velocity [65]. This suggests that PP has no adverse cerebral effects in patients with no intracranial pathology. However, in patients with either head injuries or intracranial space occupying lesions, PP might cause a dangerous rise in ICP.

Special monitoring and therapeutic measures should be considered when a laparoscopic procedure is planned for a patient with a known increased ICP.

Monitoring

When patients with intracranial lesions are schedule for laparoscopic procedures, continual monitoring of the CVP and blood CO_2 levels is recommended. A significant rise in either of these two parameters may indirectly indicate a rise in ICP.

If a patient arrives in the operating room with signs of increased ICP, continuous ICP monitoring is recommended during laparoscopy. Fiberoptic ICP pressure transducers that can be inserted intracranially through a 2.5-mm hole in the skull are now commercially available.

Prevention and Treatment

Since an elevated ICP may compromise cerebral blood flow, all efforts should be made to avoid a further rise in ICP in patients with intracranial pathology. The CVP and arterial PCO_2 should be maintained in the lower normal range. This can be accomplished by tightly controlling intravenous fluid administration and using diuretics and vasodilators for the former, and by moderately hyperventilating the lungs for the latter.

All vasodilators reduce CVP; however, nitroglycerine [66] and nitroprusside [67] may increase ICP and, therefore, should be avoided in patients with increased ICP. In contrast, trimetaphan, a ganglion blocker, promotes vasodilation without causing a significant increase in ICP [68]. This drug, therefore, is the vasodilator of choice for patients with increased ICP.

On occasion, patients sustain hypercarbia during laparoscopy (see above). Since CO_2 is a potent cerebral vasodilator, special attention should be paid to the blood CO_2 level during laparoscopy in patients with increased ICP.

References

1. Holohan TV (1991) Laparoscopic cholecystectomy. Lancet 338:801–803
2. Schirmer BD, Edge SB, Dix J, Hyser H, Banks JB, Scott Jones R (1990) Laparoscopic cholecystectomy. Treatment of choice for symptomatic cholelithiosis. Am Surg. 213(6):665–677
3. Kent RB (1991) Subcutaneous emphysema and hypercarbia following laparoscopic cholecystectomy. Arch Surg 126:1154–1156
4. Schauer PR, Sirinek KR (1994) The laparoscopic approach reduces the endocrine response to elective cholecystectomy. Am Surg 61(2):106–111
5. Volz J, Koster S, Weiss M et al (1996) Pathophysiologic features of pneumoperitoneum at laparoscopy: a swine model. Am J Obstet Gynecol 174:132–140
6. Sha M, Ohnura A, Yamada M (1991) Diaphragm function and pulmonary complications after laparoscopic cholecystectomy. Anesthesiology 75[Suppl 3A]:A255
7. Wittgen CM, Andrus CH, Fitzgerald SD et al (1991) Analysis of the hemodynamic and ventilatory effects of laparoscopic cholecystectomy. Arch Surg 126:997–1000
8. Ciofolo MJ, Clergue F, Seebacher J et al (1990) Ventilatory effects of laparoscopy under epidural anesthesia. Anesth Analg 70:357–361
9. Puri GD, Singh H (1992) Ventilatory effects of laparoscopy under general anesthesia. Br J Anaesth 68:211–213
10. Joris JL, Noirot DP, Legrand MJ et al (1993) Hemodynamic changes during laparoscopic cholecystectomy. Anesth Analg 76:1067–1071
11. Richardson JD, Trinkli EK (1976) Hemodynamic and respiratory alterations with increased intraabdominal pressure. J Surg Res 20:401–404
12. Lenz RJ, Thomas TA, Wilkins DG (1976) Cardiovascular changes during laparoscopy: studies of stroke volume and cardiac output using impedance cardiography. Anaesthesia 31:4–12
13. McKenzie R, Wadhwa R, Bedger R (1980) Noninvasive measurement of cardiac output during laparoscopy. J Reprod Med 24:247–250
14. Beebe DS, McNevin MP, Belani KG et al (1992) Evidence of venous stasis after abdominal insufflation for laparoscopic cholecystectomy. Anesthesiology 77[Suppl 3A]:A148
15. Cunningham AJ, Turner J, Rosenbaum S, Rafferty T (1993) Transesophageal assessment of haemodynamic function during laparoscopic cholecystectomy. Br J Anaesth 70:621–625
16. Ivankovich AD, Miletich DJ, Albrecht RF et al (1975) Cardiovascular effects of intraperitoneal insufflation with carbon dioxide and nitrous oxide in the dog. Anesthesiology 42:281–287

17. Versichelen L, Serreyn R, Rolly G, Vanderkerckhove D (1984) Pathophysiologic changes during anesthesia administration for gynecologic laparoscopy. J Reprod Med 29:697–700

18. Diamant M, Benumof JL, Saidman LJ (1978) Hemodynamics of increased intra-abdominal pressure: interaction with hypovolemia and halothane anesthesia. Anesthesiology 48:23–27

19. Marshall RL, Jebson PJR, Davie IT, Scott DB (1972) Circulatory effects of peritoneal insufflation with nitrous oxide. Br J Anaesth 44:1183–1187

20. Solis-Herruzo JA, Moreno D, Gonzales (1991) Effect of intrathoracic pressure on plasma arginine vasopressin levels. Gastroenterology 101:607–617

21. Joris JL, Lamy M (1993) Neuroendocrine changes during pneumoperitoneum for laparoscopic cholecystectomy. Br J Anaesth 70:A33

22. Harman PK, Kron IL, McLachlan HD (1982) Elevated intra-abdominal pressure and renal function. Ann Surg 196:594–597

23. Richards MO, Scovill W, Shin B, Reed W (1983) Acute renal failure associated with increased intra-abdominal pressure. Ann Surg 197:183–187

24. Caldwell CB, Ricotta JJ (1987) Changes in visceral blood flow with elevated intraabdominal pressure. J Surg Res 43:14–20

25. Chiu AW, Chang LS, Birkett DH, Babayan RK (1995) The impact of pneumoperitoneum and pneumoretroperitoneum and gasless laparoscopy on the systemic and renal hemodynamics. J Am Coll Surg 181:397–406

26. Blobner M, Felber AR, Gogler S et al (1992) Carbon dioxide uptake from peritoneum during laparoscopic cholecystectomy. Anesthesiology 77[Suppl 3A]:A37

27. Seed RF, Shakespeare TF, Muldoon MJ (1970) Carbon dioxide homeostasis during anaesthesia for laparoscopy. Anaesthesia 25:223–231

28. Wilcox S, Vandam LD (1988) Alas, poor Trendelenburg and his position! Anesth Analg 67:574–578

29. Batra MS, Driscoll JJ, Coburn WA, Marks WM (1983) Evanescent nitrous oxide pneumothorax after laparoscopy. Anesth Analg 62:1121–1123

30. Whiston RJ, Eggers KA, Movus RW, Stamatakis JD (1991) Tension pneumothorax during laparoscopic cholecystectomy. Br J Surg 78:1325

31. Phillips JM, Keith D, Hulka J et al (1976) Gynecologic laparoscopy in 1975. J Reprod Med 16:105–117

32. Gomar C, Fernandez C, Villalonga A, Nalda MA (1985) Carbon dioxide embolism during laparoscopy and hysteroscopy. Ann Fr Anesth Reanim 4:380–382

33. Diakun TA (1991) Carbon dioxide embolism: successful resuscitation with cardiopulmonary bypass. Anesthesiology 74:1151–1153

34. Morison DH, Riggs JRA (1974) Cardiovascular collapse in laparoscopy. Can Med Assoc J 111:433–437

35. Nichols SL, Tompkins BM, Henderson PA (1981) Probable carbon dioxide embolism during laparoscopy; case report. Wis Med J 80:27–29

36. Shulman D, Aronson HB (1984) Capnography in the early diagnosis of CO_2 embolism during laparoscopy. Can J Anaesth 31:455–459

37. De Plater RM, Jones ISC (1989) Non-fatal carbon dioxide embolism during laparoscopy. Anaesth Intensive Care 17:359–361

38. McGrath BJ, Zimmerman JE, Williams JF, Parmet J (1989) Carbon dioxide embolism treated with hyperbaric oxygen. Can J Anaesth 36:586–589

39. Ostman PL, Pantle-Fisher FH, Faure EA, Glosten B (1990) Circulatory collapse during laparoscopy. J Clin Anesth 2:129–132

40. Yacoub OF, Cadona L, Coveler LA, Dodson MG (1982) Carbon dioxide embolism during laparoscopy. Anesthesiology 57:533–535

41. Brantley JC, Riley PM (1988) Cardiovascular collapse during laparoscopy: a report of two cases. Am J Obstet Gynecol 159:735–737

42. Perry PM, Baughman VL (1990) A complication of laparoscopy: air embolism. Anesthesiology 73:546–547

43. Greville AC, Clements AF, Erwin DC et al (1991) Pulmonary air embolism during laparoscopic laser cholecystectomy. Anaesthesia 46:113–114

44. Root B, Levy MN, Pollack S et al (1978) Gas embolism death after laparoscopy in the portal circulation. Anesth Analg 57:232–237

45. Schroder TM, Puolakkainen PA, Hahl J, Ramo OJ (1989) Fatal air embolism as a complication of laser-induced hyperthermia. Laser Surg Med 9:183–185
46. Baggish MS, Daniell JF (1989) Catastrophic injury secondary to the use of coaxial gas-cooled fibers and artificial sapphire tips for intrauterine surgery: a report of five cases. Laser Surg Med 9:581–584
47. Graff TD, Arbegast NR, Phillips OC et al (1959) Gas embolism; a comparative study of air and CO_2 as embolic agents in the systemic venous system. Am J Obstet Gynecol 78:259
48. Hagen PT, Scholtz DG, Edwards WD (1984) Incidence and size of patent foramen ovale during the first 10 decades of life: an autopsy study of 965 normal hearts. Mayo Clin Proc 59:17–20
49. Khan MA, Alkalay I, Suetsugu S, Stein M (1972) Acute changes in lung mechanics following pulmonary emboli of various gases in dogs. J Appl Physiol 33:774–777
50. English JB, Westenskow D, Hodges MR, Stanley TH (1978) Comparison of venous air embolism monitoring methods in supine dog. Anesthesiology 48:425–429
51. Desai S, Roaf E, Liu P (1982) Acute pulmonary edema during laparoscopy. Anesth Analg 61:699–700
52. Wadhwa RK, McKenzie R, Wadhwa SR et al (1978) Gas embolism during laparoscopy. Anesthesiology 48:74–76
53. Tay HS, Chiu HH (1989) Acid aspiration during laparoscopy. Anaesth Intensive Care 6:134–136
54. Duffy BL (1979) Regurgitation during pelvic laparoscopy. Br J Anaesth 51:1089–1090
55. Jones MJ, Mitchell RW, Hindocha N et al (1989) Effect of increased intra-abdominal pressure during laparoscopy on the lower esophageal sphincter. Anesth Analg 68:63–65
56. Heijke SA, Smith G, Key A (1991) The effect of the Trendelenburg position on the lower oesophageal sphincter tone. Anaesthesia 46:185–187
57. Bernhard WN, Cottrell JE, Silvakumaran C et al (1979) Adjustment of intracuff pressure to prevent aspiration. Anesthesiology 50:363–366
58. Hamelberg W, Bosomworth PP (1964) Aspiration pneumonitis: experimental studies and clinical observations. Anesth Analg 43:669–670
59. Lewis DG, Ryder W, Burn N et al (1972) Laparoscopy – an investigation during spontaneous ventilation with halothane. Br J Anaesth 44:685–691
60. Carmichael DE (1971) Laparoscopy-cardiac considerations. Fertil Steril 22:69–70
61. Harris MN, Plantevin OM, Crowther A (1984) Cardiac arrhythmia during anaesthesia for laparoscopy. Br J Anaesth 56:1213–1217
62. Kenefick JP, Leader A, Maltby JR, Taylor PJ (1987) Laparoscopy: blood-gas values and minor sequelae associated with three techniques based on isoflurane. Br J Anaesth 59:189–194
63. Josephs LG, Este-McDonald JR, Birkett DH, Hirsch EF (1994) Diagnostic laparoscopy increases intracranial pressure. J Trauma 36:815–818
64. Harper AM, Glass HI (1965) Effect of elevations in arterial carbon dioxide tension on the blood flow through the cerebral cortex at normal and low arterial blood pressures. J Neurol Neurosurg Psychiatry 28:449–455
65. Kirkinen P, Hirvonen E, Kauko M et al (1995) Intracranial blood flow during laparoscopic hysterectomy. Acta Obstet Gynecol Scand 74:71–74
66. Ghani GA, Sung YF, Weinstein MS et al (1983) Effects of intravenous nitroglycerine on the intracranial pressure and volume pressure response. J Neurosurg 58:562–565
67. Griswold WR, Reznik V, Mendoza SA (1981) Nitroprusside-induced intracranial hypertension (letter). JAMA 246:2679–80
68. Turner JM, Powell D, McDowall DG (1977) Intracranial pressure changes in neurosurgical patients during hypotension induced with sodium nitroprusside or trimetaphan. Br J Anaesth 49:419–425
69. Rosenthal RJ, Hiatt JR, Phillips EH, Hewitt W, Demetriou AA, Grode M (1997) Effects of pneumoperitoneum on intracranial pressure. Large animal model observations. Surg Endosc 11: 376–380
70. Irgau, Koyfman Y, Tikelis JL (1995) Elective intraoperative intracranial pressure monitoring during laparoscopic cholecystectomy. Arch Surg, 130: 1011–1013
71. Joris JL (1994) Anesthetic management of laparoscopy. In: Miller RD (ed) Anesthesia, 4th edn. Churchill Livingstone, New York
72. Joris J, Ledoux D, Honorei* P, Lamy M (1991) Ventilatory effects of CO_2 insufflation during laparoscopic cholecystectomy. Anesthesiology 75[Suppl 3A]:A121

13 Pneumoperitoneum-Related Complications: Diagnosis and Treatment

A.S. LOWHAM, C.J. FILIPI, and T. TOMONAGA

Introduction

Technological advances and the innovations of many laparoscopic surgeons have resulted in a rapid expansion of diagnostic and therapeutic laparoscopy. Experience has demonstrated that adequate exposure of the operative field is critical in the performance of successful laparoscopic surgery. Currently, the development of a carbon dioxide pneumoperitoneum in combination with patient positioning and appropriate retraction are the preferred methods of obtaining consistent and safe exposure.

This chapter explores complications associated with the development and maintenance of a pneumoperitoneum during laparoscopic surgery. These may include trocar injuries, subcutaneous emphysema, gas embolism, venous stasis, and cardiorespiratory changes. The diagnosis, treatment, and prevention of iatrogenic, physiologic, and functional pneumoperitoneum-related complications are discussed.

Pneumoperitoneum Agents

Historically, a number of gases have been used to facilitate diagnostic and therapeutic laparoscopy. The ideal insufflation gas would be inexpensive, readily available, physiologically inert, nonexplosive in the presence of coagulation, and capable of rapid pulmonary excretion. Insufflation gases used in addition to carbon dioxide have included air, oxygen, nitrous oxide, and helium.

In 1933 Fervers documented the first case of an intra-abdominal explosion while using 100% O_2 as the insufflating gas [1]. Nitrous oxide (N_2O) has been implicated in two case reports of intra-abdominal explosions during laparoscopic female sterilization in the 1970s [2, 3]. Despite concerns about its potential for combustion, monopolar and bipolar tubal sterilization have been safely performed in hundreds of thousands of cases using N_2O pneumoperitoneum. The potential hazard of N_2O results from the concurrent presence of hydrogen or methane in sufficient concentrations (5.5% and 4%, respectively) to support combustion [4]. Hunter demonstrated the highest measured concentration of hydrogen to be 70 times less than that threshold and the detection of no methane in 20 clinical laparoscopies [4]. Despite this, concerns over the escape of sufficient hydrogen or methane from an unrecognized bowel perforation and the development of an explosion hazard have limited its use. Of note, Neuman demonstrated that when N_2O is used as an inhalation anesthetic, it can reach sufficient concentrations in the peritoneal cavity (47%) during laparoscopy with a CO_2 pneumoperitoneum to conceivably support combustion if a sufficient amount of methane or hydrogen from a bowel perforation were present [5].

Helium has also been investigated as a possible alternative. Leighton compared the cardiopulmonary effects of CO_2 and helium pneumoperitoneum. In contrast to CO_2, helium pneumoperitoneum did not result in hypercarbia, acidemia, or pulmonary hypertension [6]. Helium possesses other desirable characteristics including availability, low cost, and rapid excretion from pulmonary arterial blood into the alveoli with virtually no retention in the systemic circulation. Concerns, however, arise over the lower aqueous solubility of helium compared to CO_2. Although this is beneficial by resulting in less absorption from the peritoneal cavity, if helium gas embolism occurs its low solubility may result in persistence of gas bubbles. Nonetheless, helium is highly diffusible and it is proposed that this may aid in the dissolution of helium emboli [6].

Although carbon dioxide is the current insufflating gas of choice, insufflation of CO_2 into the peritoneal cavity can result in serious hypercarbia caused in part by the absorption of gas across the peritoneal surface. The ensuing respiratory acidosis and acidemia can contribute to arrhythmias and alterations in cardiac hemodynamics.

Trocar Insertion

Visceral and major vessel injury by needle or primary trocar insertion for the creation of a pneumoperitoneum remains a problem in laparoscopic surgery. Injuries sustained using either the closed or open technique represent a preventable cause of morbidity. The closed technique utilizes a spring-loaded needle with a blunt obturator developed by Janos Veress in 1938. The Veress needle retracts during penetration of the abdominal wall and springs forward upon fascial penetration to prevent visceral injury. A second blind insertion is performed to place the primary trocar. No viable method exists to ascertain the position of underlying vital structures prior to blind insertion of the needle or trocar. The incidence of blood vessel or gastrointestinal tract injury during insertion of the Veress needle or primary trocar is estimated to be 0.2% [7], with the majority of major vascular injuries during laparoscopy resulting from the insertion of needles or trocars for creation of the pneumoperitoneum [8]. In addition, some injuries previously ascribed to electrosurgical techniques may actually be the result of trocar insertion [9]. Preventive measures to minimize potential complications during closed laparoscopy include elevation of the fascia prior to needle insertion, aspiration to rule out blood vessel penetration, the "hanging drop test" (the needle water column drops secondary to negative pressure), thus verifying an intraperitoneal position of the needle tip, and a full pneumoperitoneum prior to blind insertion of the primary trocar. Other precautions include directing the trocar into the pelvis rather than simply posteriorly and positioning the inserting-hand index finger parallel to the trocar, preventing deep trocar penetration into the peritoneal cavity.

The open technique described by Hasson in 1971 utilizes a fascial incision followed by direct incision or forceps penetration of the peritoneum [10]. Others favor direct trocar penetration to enter the peritoneal cavity [11]. Although the incidence of major vascular injury has decreased, the incidence of visceral injury has remained unchanged with wider use of the open technique [12].

In an effort to reduce intraperitoneal injury, trocars have been designed with blunt tips or protective sheaths that enclose the trocar blade after peritoneal entry. Other innovations include new "optical trocars" that allow visualization of the layers of the abdominal wall as the trocar is inserted. The laparoscope is inserted into the trocar itself prior to insertion.

Veress-needle injury of the bowel is best managed by leaving the needle in the viscera followed by laparoscopic suturing or laparotomy. Secondary trocar

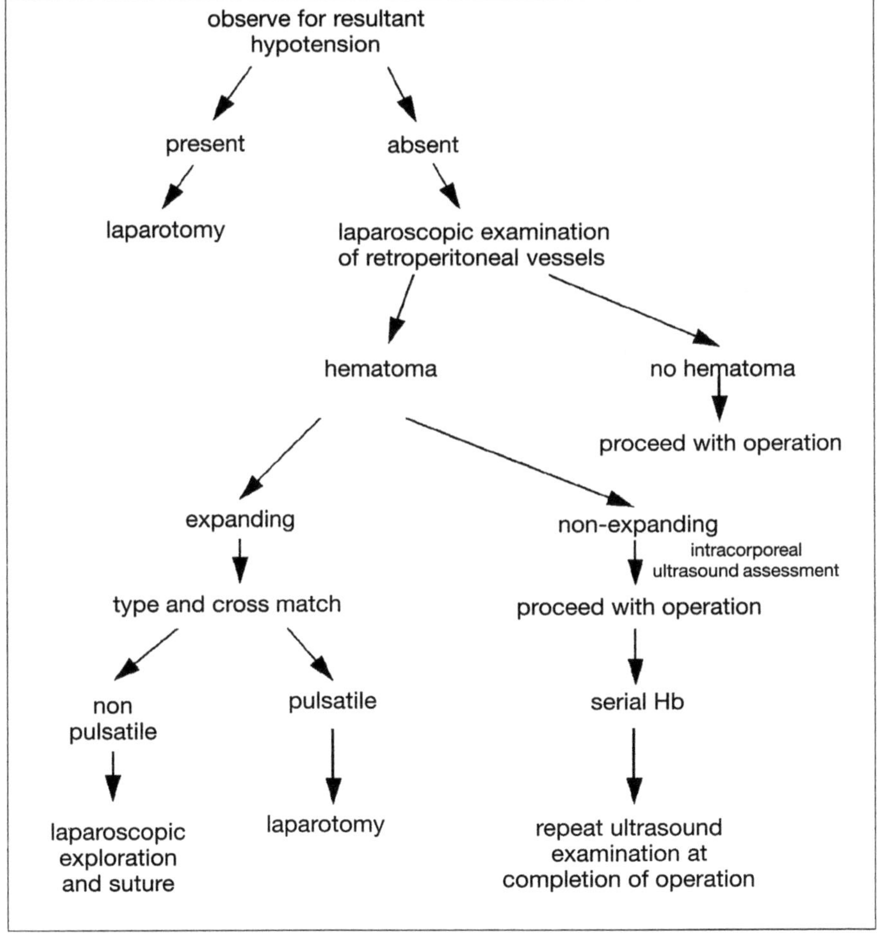

Fig. 1. Suspected Veress needle injury of major vessel

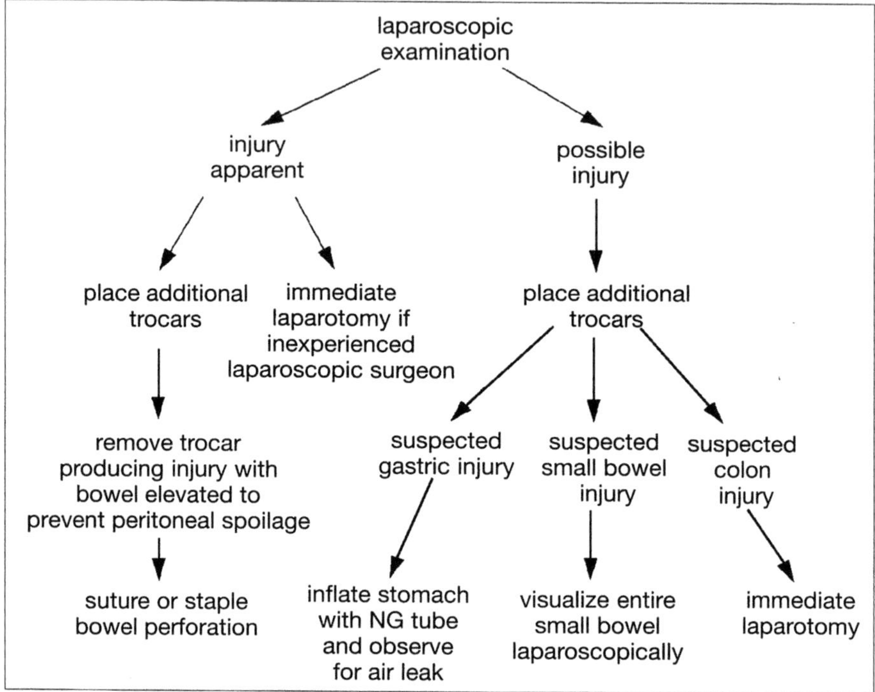

Fig. 2. Suspected primary trocar injury of bowel

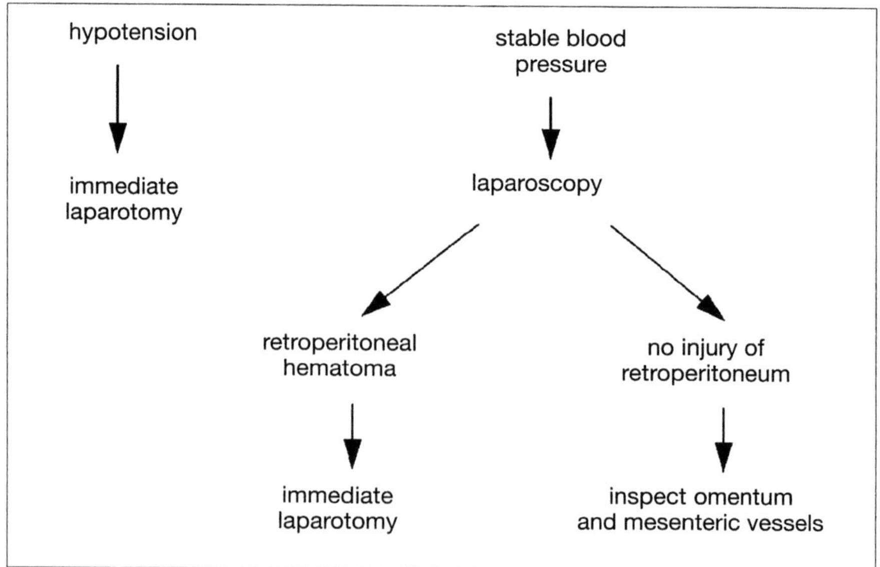

Fig. 3. Suspected primary trocar injury of major vessel

injuries to the gastrointestinal tract can be assessed for laparoscopic repair. A 5-mm trocar penetration of the urinary bladder only requires foley catheter placement, while larger trocar injuries may necessitate suture closure and drainage. The algorithms in Figures 1–3 have been developed to assist in decision making.

Venous Stasis

Venous stasis is one component of Virchow's triad contributing to the formation of deep venous thrombosis (DVT) and the risk of pulmonary embolism (PE). Other factors including hypercoagulability and endothelial damage are known to be induced by operative procedures and may contribute to thrombus formation in patients undergoing laparoscopic surgery. A prospective study of 50247 patients undergoing gynecological laparoscopy revealed an incidence of 0.2 for DVT and 0.2 for PE per 1000 laparoscopies [13].

The development of a pneumoperitoneum with an intra-abdominal pressure greater than central venous pressure (CVP) reduces venous flow from the lower extremities through compression of the inferior vena cava (IVC). This results in reduced pulsatility in the femoral venous system [14] and a significant increase in femoral venous diameter [15]. The placement of patients in the reverse-Trendelenburg position, common during laparoscopic cholecystectomy and many upper abdominal laparoscopies such as fundoplication, may also act to inhibit venous return [16]. In addition, longer, more complicated laparoscopic procedures are being performed which may also act to increase the risk of DVT.

The use of intermittent sequential pneumatic compression stockings has been shown to return peak systolic velocity in the femoral veins to normal [16, 17]. The prophylactic use of sequential stockings addresses one component of Virchow's triad-venous stasis and is recommended for all laparoscopies. A transient hypercoagulable state has also been demonstrated after laparoscopic cholecystectomy and the selective use of postoperative heparin is recommended [18].

Hemodynamics

Adverse physiologic effects resulting from pneumoperitoneum are related to both hypercarbia and the mechanical effects of increased abdominal pressure and patient positioning. Physiologic events resulting from carbon dioxide pneumoperitoneum are especially important with the expansion of laparoscopic surgery and its use on more elderly patients, often with significant co-morbid conditions.

Hypercarbia is partially related to transperitoneal absorption of CO_2 and results in an elevated PCO_2 and end-tidal CO_2 ($ETCO_2$). Rapid peritoneal distention secondary to pneumoperitoneum may induce an exaggerated vagal response resulting in bradycardia and cardiovascular collapse. Intra-abdominal hypertension increases afterload, venous resistance, and mean systemic pressure. The increased afterload results from mechanical compression of the splanchnic circulation. Increased venous resistance results from compression of the IVC and decreasing venous return. In contrast, the increase in mean systemic pressure resulting from compression of the capacitance vessels acts as a pump to increase venous return and is a component of preload. In hyopovolemic or euvolemic patients the influence of increased venous resistance predominates and venous return is decreased with pneumoperitoneum. In hypervolemic patients, the influence of increased systemic pressure predominates with minimal compression of the IVC, resulting in increased venous return [19, 20].

In a swine model Ortega noted a decrease in IVC flow by 24% at 5 min and 31% at 60 min after initiation of a 15 mmHg CO_2 pneumoperitoneum. They noted a paradoxic increase in cardiac output and stroke volume without an associated tachycardia [19]. Marathe demonstrated in dogs that an intra-abdominal pressure (IAP) greater than 15 mmHg resulted in a decrease in cardiac output and left ventricular (LV) end-diastolic volume, but no change in mean arterial pres-

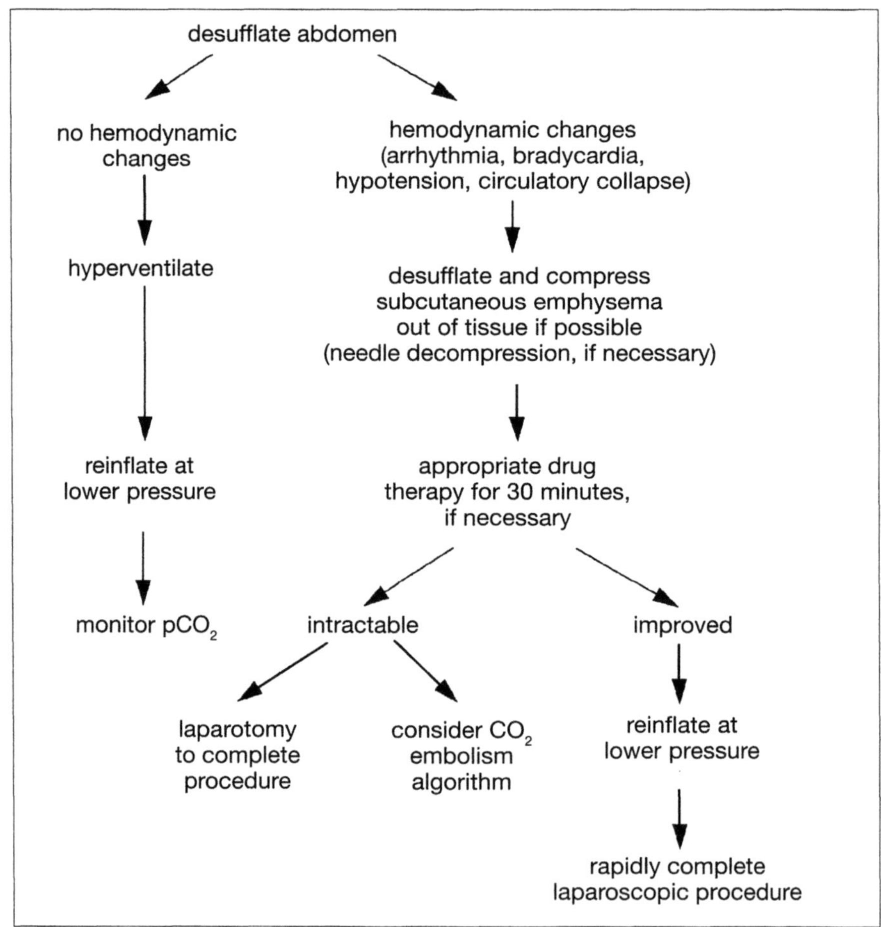

Fig. 4. Confirmed acidosis during laparoscopic surgery

sure (MAP), heart rate or LV contractility with an IAP of 5–25 mmHg. They concluded that hemodynamic alterations of CO_2 pneumoperitoneum were related to altered LV preload and not alterations in contractility or LV afterload [21].

In human subjects undergoing laparoscopic surgery with a 15-mmHg pneumoperitoneum, McLaughlin demonstrated a significant increase in MAP (15.9%), systolic blood pressure (11.3%), diastolic blood pressure (19.7%), and CVP (30%). In addition, decreases in stroke volume (29.5%) and cardiac index (29.5%) were noted [22]. Westerband also studied human subjects undergoing laparoscopic cholecystectomy with a 15-mmHg pneumoperitoneum. A decrease in cardiac output (30%), increased MAP (15%), and total peripheral vascular resistance (79%) were noted. The elevation in afterload may increase the myocardial oxygen consumption and the possibility of myocardial infarction in susceptible patients [23, 24]. Concerns over the mechanical effects of high pneumoperitoneum pressures have led to investigation into the ideal pressure. Ishizaki has demonstrated that some hemodynamic effects including a decreased cardiac output and elevated systemic vascular resistance occurring with a 16-mmHg pneumoperitoneum were not present with an 8- or 12-mmHg pneumoperitoneum [25]. Patients at risk should undergo careful perioperative hemodynamic monitoring to reduce the possibility of cardiac morbidity.

Changes in pulmonary physiology are also primarily related to mechanical effects of the pneumoperitoneum. The increase in intra-abdominal volume and pressure results in decreased diaphragmatic excursion with a rise in intrathoracic and peak airway pressure, and a decrease in pulmonary compliance and vital capacity. Most respiratory effects related to pneumoperitoneum in current laparoscopy are limited and easily compensated for by an increase in tidal volume or respiratory rate.

Laparoscopists and anesthesia personnel must be aware of the variable hemodynamic alterations which may be induced by CO_2 pneumoperitoneum. The algorithm shown in Figure 4 is a guideline for the assessment of hemodynamic changes during laparoscopy.

Carbon Dioxide Gas Embolism

The mechanism and true incidence of gas embolism during laparoscopy are unknown. Philips reported 15 instances of gas embolism during 113|523 gynecologic laparoscopies [26]. Although multiple cases of significant gas embolism during gynecologic laparoscopy have been reported (Table 1) [27–36], only one case of fatal CO_2 gas embolism during laparoscopic upper abdominal surgery including cholecystectomy has been reported [27]. Using end-tidal capnography and precordial Doppler ultrasound on 61 consecutive patients undergoing laparoscopic biliary procedures, Landercasper was unable to detect evidence of gas embolization [37]. In contrast, Derouin performed transesophageal echocardiography (TEE) and detected CO_2 embolism in 10 of 15 patients undergoing laparoscopic cholecystectomy. All events occurred without a change in cardiorespiratory status [38].

Despite the rarity of CO_2 embolism, it represents a potentially fatal event and rapid intervention must be initiated. To produce a significant cardiorespiratory

Table 1. Case reports of carbon dioxide embolism during laparoscopy

Reference	Case no	IAP mm Hg	Method of Insufflation	Time to symptoms from initial insufflation	Signs/symptoms	Outcome
[27]	1	13	Veress	3 min insufflation	Bradycardia, CV collapse, mydriasis, mill wheel murmur	Death Death
	2	10	Veress	During insufflation	Cyanosis, bradycardia, CV collapse	
	3	15	NA	During insufflation	Bradycardia, coma, status epilepticus	
	4	14	NA	During insufflation	Cyanosis, vent. arryth., mydriasis, mill wheel murmur	
	5	13	NA	During	Bradycardia	
	6	12	NA	10 min	CV collapse, mill wheel murmur	
	7	10	NA	During insufflation	Bradycardia, hypertension	
[28]	8	15	NA	60 min	Decreased $ETCO_2$, CV collapse, mill wheel murmur	Death
[29]	9	NA	Veress	35 min	CV collapse, increased $ETCO_2$	
[30]	10	NA	NA	55 min	Decreased $ETCO_2$, cyanosis	
[31]	11	10–20	Veress	During insufflation	CV collapse, decreased $ETCO_2$, mill wheel murmur	
[32]	12	NA	Veress	35 min	Bradycardia, Cyanosis	
[33]	13	10–20	Veress	Early	CV collapse, mill wheel murmur	
[34]	14	NA	Veress	35 min	Cyanosis, CV collapse	Death
[35]	15	10–20	Veress	During	Bradycardia, CV collapse, mill wheel murmur	
[36]	16	> 30	Veress	Early	Cyanosis, CV collapse	
	17	> 30	Veress	Early	Bradycardia, CV collapse	

IAP = Intraabdominal pressure; CV, cardiovascular; $ETCO_2$, end tidal carbon dioxide;
NA = Not available

event a large amount of CO_2 must enter the venous circulation with mechanical occlusion of the right heart or outflow tract of the right ventricle. Impaired venous return and cor pulmonale result in elevated central venous pressure, hypoxia, dysrhymthias, and LV failure. Case reports indicate most episodes of significant gas embolism manifest as bradycardia, cyanosis, and rapid cardiovascular collapse (Table 1) [27–36]. A characteristic loud churning "mill wheel" murmur audible without a stethoscope has been described, while others report only a coarse systolic murmur [39, 40]. An acute drop in $ETCO_2$ has also been proposed as a diagnostic tool, although a rise in $ETCO_2$ has been noted in some cases [41]. In describing seven cases of "gas embolism" with two deaths during laparoscopy, Cottin described bradycardia and cardiovascular collapse as the presenting signs in five patients, while cyanosis was the initial manifestation in two. In addition, bilateral mydriasis was found in five patients. All cases occurred on insufflation or soon after, and all patients had undergone previous abdominal or pelvic surgery. Note that direct cardiac aspiration did not prove the diagnosis in these instances of circulatory failure [27] and post mortem diagnosis may not be obtainable due to the high solubility of CO_2.

Dion compared the hemodynamic effects in dogs of an intravenous bolus injection of CO_2 versus a 1-cm venotomy in the infrarenal IVC of dogs with a 12- to 15-mmHg pneumoperitoneum. A Swan Ganz catheter was placed for hemodynamic monitoring and TEE was used to assess for the presence of CO_2 bubbles. With a 12–15-mmHg pneumoperitoneum and the venotomy, TEE detected CO_2 bubbles in the right atrium and ventricle in only two of 11 instances without hemodynamic changes, including elevation of pulmonary artery pressure (PAP). In 15 instances, a 15-cc intravenous bolus of CO_2 was given and detected by TEE but without significant change in PAP. With the intravenous injection of 100 cc CO_2 a significant elevation of PAP occurred when compared to dogs submitted to venotomy or injected with 15 cc CO_2. Finally, a massive bolus injection of 300 cc CO_2 led to the appearance of fused gas bubbles in the left ventricle and death in all dogs [42].

In 1947, Durant described the left lateral position as an effective treatment to release the "gas lock" in the pulmonary outflow tract [39]. Subsequently, Michenfelder popularized intracardiac aspiration as a treatment [40]. Comparative studies of these methods, as well as cardiac massage to fragment the air and encourage its distribution into smaller branches of the pulmonary arterial tree, demonstrated equal effectiveness [43]. Diakun reported placing a patient on cardiopulmonary bypass following circulatory collapse during simultaneous laparoscopy and hysteroscopy. A gas lock was noted in the right atrium causing obstruction of the IVC. Subsequent venting released gas from all four chambers with eventual patient recovery [29].

The most likely etiologies of gas embolism during laparoscopy include venous injury during laparoscopic dissection or inadvertent placement of the Veress needle into a vessel during initial insufflation. It is notable that in approximately two thirds of cases, signs of gas embolism are evident during or immediately following insufflation, while the remaining cases have occurred 10–55 min after initial insufflation (Table 1) [27–36]. When specified, all cases of CO_2 embolism have taken place with use of the Veress needle [27, 29, 31–36]. Careful placement of the Veress needle into the peritoneal cavity, in addition to aspiration to rule out blood vessel placement, is necessary. Neglect of aspiration, especially when repeated attempts at needle placement are required, can lead to this life-threatening complication.

If a CO_2 embolus is suspected, the patient should be placed in the left lateral, head-down position if possible, insufflation stopped, the pneumoperitoneum released, 100% oxygen supplied, dysrhymthias management initiated, and closed-chest compressions performed. Venous catheters may be placed for superior vena cava (SVC), right atrial, ventricle, and outflow tract aspiration. In the event of refractory cardiac arrest, cardiopulmonary bypass may be considered [41]. The administration of N_2O as an anesthetic agent should be stopped since it rapidly

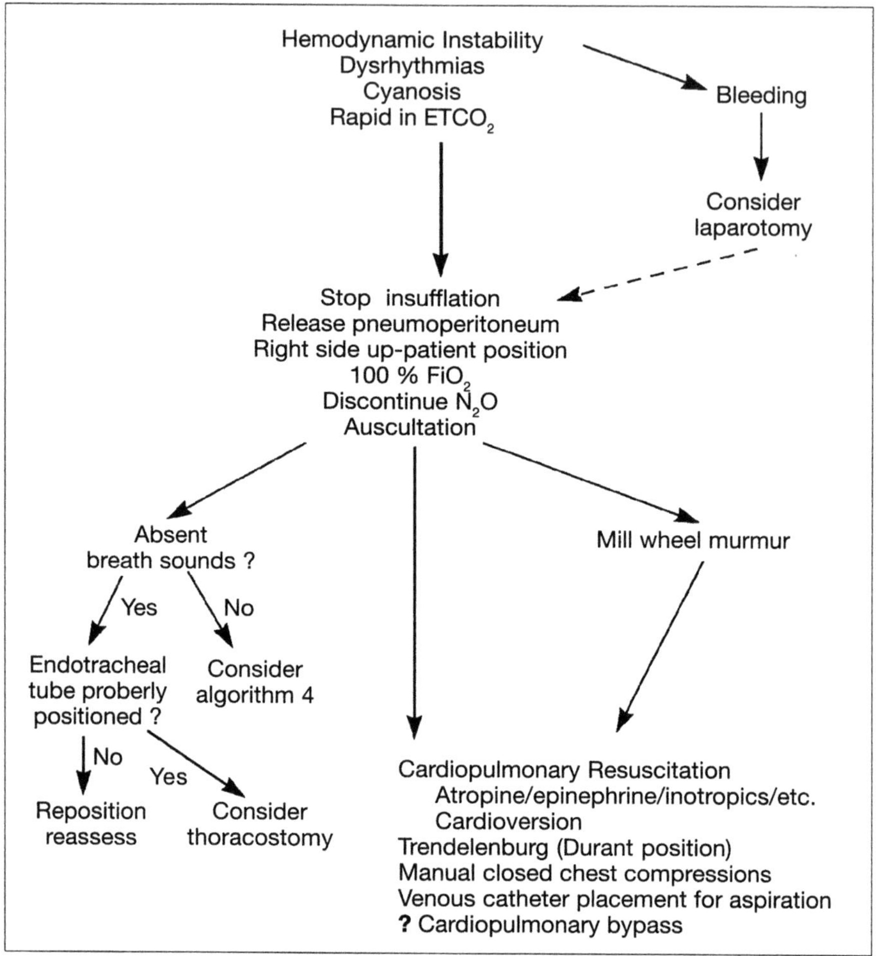

Fig. 5.   Gas embolism

enters the gas space containing CO_2, thus adding to the gas volume [44]. Figure 5 summarizes the therapeutic management of cases of suspected gas embolism.

Pneumothorax, Subcutaneous Emphysema, and Pneumomediastinum

The development of a pneumothorax during laparoscopic surgery may arise from various mechanisms. The incidence of pneumothorax was reported by Loffer to be 0.1/1000 cases in gynecological laparoscopy [45]. A review of 70 reported cases revealed a predominance of right-sided pneumothorax (79%) and five cases of tension pneumothorax with death in two patients [46]. The first reports occurred with the use of pneumoperitoneum to treat tuberculous ascites. Mellies demonstrated free movement of fluid between the right thoracic cavity and abdominal cavity in the case of a spontaneous right pneumothorax with pneumoperitoneum, and Smith demonstrated multiple congenital defects in the diaphragm of a patient with fatal bilateral pneumothoraces [47, 48].

Theories have also been explored investigating the possibility of spontaneous pneumothorax resulting from the high diffusion capacity of CO_2 [49]. Prystowsky reported a spontaneous bilateral pneumothorax diagnosed radiographically during laparoscopic cholecystectomy in a healthy 21-year-old male. Laparoscopic inspection revealed no evidence of diaphragmatic defects and manual ventilation with an increased minute volume allowed completion of the surgery. Within 90 min postoperatively, the pneumothoraces had nearly completely resolved suggesting CO_2 was the space-occupying gas [46]. Iatrogenic cases are seen with the advent of laparoscopic antireflux surgery and the creation of a posterior esophageal window. If the dissection is performed above the left crus, entry into the left chest is possible with a resulting pneumothorax.

Animal studies performed by Marcus compared physiological parameters between a pneumoperitoneum and pneumoperitoneum with concurrent pneumothorax created by a laceration in the left diaphragm. The creation of a pneumoperitoneum resulted in hypoxemia ($^-pO_2$, $^-O_2$ saturation), respiratory acidosis and an increase in peak inspiratory pressure (PIP). All of these parameters were significantly exacerbated upon the creation of a pneumothorax but returned to normal with simple desufflation, increasing minute ventilation, or suturing of the diaphragmatic laceration. Although these parameters may become evident in the operating room, a tension pneumothorax is unlikely due to the equilibration between the pleural and peritoneal cavities and standard insufflation pressures (12–15 mmHg) [49]. Intraoperative findings suggesting a pneumothorax include the presence of subcutaneous emphysema, an abrupt rise in $ETCO_2$, an increase in airway pressure, decreased compliance, hypoxemia, and diminished or absent breath sounds. In addition, jugular venous distension with hypotension are seen with tension pneumothorax. Differentiation must be made from bronchial intubation resulting from initial endotracheal tube misplacement, shifting of the endotracheal tube with patient movement, or after peritoneal insufflation resulting in a cephalad shift in the diaphragm and right bronchial intubation. In these situations, hypoxemia and elevated airway pressure occur earlier in the procedure and $ETCO_2$ initially remains normal. After clinical or radiologic intraoperative diagnosis, insufflation is stopped, the pneumoperitoneum is released, and hyperventilation performed to normalize CO_2. If significant cardiorespiratory effects are present or a pneumothorax occurs early in the surgical procedure, consideration is given to tube thoracostomy [41, 46]. Most pneumothoraces are noted on postoperative radiographs and, depending on the extent of the pneumothorax and the patients clinical status, chest tube thoracostomy versus conservative treatment with serial radiographs is performed.

Subcutaneous emphysema is most often seen in the setting of a pneumothorax with a parietal pleura defect, as seen after rib fracture or with chest tube placement. During laparoscopy, subcutaneous emphysema may result from mispositioning of the Veress needle within the subcutaneous tissue during insufflation, or unrecognized retraction of the tip of the primary insufflating trocar into the subcutaneous tissue. With development of the pneumoperitoneum, gas may also infiltrate the subcutaneous tissue through any trocar site with a widened fascial defect or with trocar retraction. Insufflation into the preperitoneal space during laparoscopic hernia repair has also resulted in subcutaneous emphysema [50]. Diffusion of gas through the mediastinum may produce pneumomediastinum and emphysema in the cervical-cephalic region. This often occurs during laparoscopic antireflux surgery with dissection of the lower mediastinal tissues [41].

The clinical significance of subcutaneous emphysema lies in the development of hypercarbia to a degree not seen with pneumoperitoneum alone and is due to the larger absorption surface area [41, 51]. Thus, intraoperative indications of subcutaneous emphysema include palpable crepitus and an abrupt increase in $ETCO_2$ or PCO_2. In all cases a pneumothorax should be ruled out, ventilation increased to maintain an acceptable $ETCO_2$ or PCO_2, and the mechanism determined and corrected if possible. As in other cases of CO_2 accumulation, the use of N_2O as an anesthetic agent is terminated [41, 44]. Postoperatively, the upper airway is evaluated for possible compromise resulting from compression. Spontaneous resolution of the subcutaneous emphysema over several days is expected.

Neoplastic Seeding of Trocar Sites

Reports of cancer recurrence in ports used for specimen removal or in distant instrument ports are a leading concern in the laparoscopic management of carcinoma. Tumor formation in port sites has been reported with laparoscopy performed in the presence of ovarian, gallbladder, gastric, and colorectal carcinoma [52]. As a result, enthusiasm for the laparoscopic management of colorectal carcinoma has abated. Some authors now recommend relegation of laparoscopic colectomy for carcinoma to investigative studies alone [52].

Wound recurrence is not unique to laparoscopic surgery. Hughes reported cancer recurrence rates in standard laparotomy wounds to be 0.8%, and suggested that systemic malignant disease, present at the time of surgery, may be the predominant mechanism of wound site recurrence [53]. There are several other reports of wound site recurrence after laparotomy for colorectal cancer, including a report of six incisional recurrences by Boreham in 1958 [54].

Theories include seeding during tumor removal, microperforations allowing exfoliation of tumor cells into the peritoneum, or aerosolizing of tumor cells with the pneumoperitoneum [55–57]. The theory that the pressure gradient, or "chimney effect," resulting from the release of the pneumoperitoneum causes implantation of free peritoneal tumor cells within port sites has been investigated. An in vitro investigation by Whelan was unable to demonstrate aerosolization of a sufficient number of viable tumor cells to facilitate growth [58]. Knolmayer increased a pneumoperitoneum pressure in swine from 8 mmHg to 18 mmHg by 2-mmHg increments every 30 min, while a 14-gauge angiocath placed into the peritoneum and attached to a closed system was used to collect aerosolized cells. Epithelial cells were evident at each level of pneumoperitoneum with a moderate correlation between the pressure level and the number of cells collected. A maximum of nine cells was seen at 12 mmHg [59]. Hubens demonstrated that a pneumoperitoneum did not enhance the implantation of free intraperitoneal cancer cells on the parietal peritoneum (carcinomatosis), but suggested that ports alter the topography of the carcinomatosis with implantation during deflation and trocar removal [60]. Wexner cited 44 cases of port site recurrence after laparoscopic colectomy, including 12 patients with Duke's B lesions and three with Duke's A lesions [55]. Confusion exists because some Duke's classifications categorize Stage B as tumor growth through the bowel wall into perirectal fat, while other classifications categorize B1 as limited to the muscularis propria [61]. This is an important factor because in the presence of a cancer penetrating the bowel wall with or without involvement of adjacent tissues, the etiology of port site recurrence is likely direct tumor spread with instruments or aerosolization. One recurrence in a Duke's A cancer occurred after a laparoscopic colotomy with laparoscopic stapling of the tumor pedicle and specimen removal through a right iliac trocar site. Despite clear margins of resection, the patient experienced a recurrence 9 months postoperatively at a remote trocar site. In this case, a previous attempt at colonoscopic removal, as well as tumor manipulation during the laparoscopy, may have resulted in significant exfoliation of tumor cells [62]. Laparoscopic segmental resection of an early-stage colorectal cancer would not seem to predispose to recurrence through improper manipulation or pneumoperitoneum.

Wound irrigation with cytotoxic agents, excision of trocar sites, and gasless laparoscopy have all been suggested as possible solutions [60]. In addition, releasing the pneumoperitoneum prior to trocar removal should prevent the implantation of tumor cells with desufflation. This would require direct closure of fascial defects and obviate the use of intraperitoneal fascial closure devices. Tumor implantation from intraperitoneal cancer cells located on the outer surface of the trocar is still possible upon removal.

Further studies on the mechanisms of port site recurrence and continued data collection are required. The overall incidence of this complication, especially its relation to tumor stage, is important. Although the exact etiology of port site recurrence remains unclear, avoidance of unnecessary tumor manipulation, collection bags for specimen removal, and the use of wound protectors is recommended.

Conclusion

An understanding of potential complications related to the use of pneumoperitoneum during laparoscopic surgery is necessary. Most episodes of altered cardiovascular hemodynamics during laparoscopy are self-limited and related to alterations produced by the mechanical effects of pneumoperitoneum. Rare episodes of more serious cardiovascular collapse may be related to the phenomenon of gas embolism and algorithms may assist in the appropriate assessment and response.

Concerns related to the practice of laparoscopy also include the potential hazards possible with the use of insufflating needles and trocars. Caution must be exercised with the use of these devices in all instances. Newer concerns including trocar site implantation with tumor require more study but must be considered when planning a laparoscopic approach to patient management.

References

1. Fervers C (1933) Die Laparoskopie mit dem Cystokop. Med Klin 29:1042–1045
2. El-Kady AA, Abd-El-Razek M (1976) Intraperitoneal explosion during female sterilization by laparoscopic electrocoagulation. Int J Gynaecol Obstet 14:487–488
3. Gunatilake DE (1978) Case report: fatal intraperitoneal explosion during electrocoagulation via laparoscopy. Int J Gynaecol Obstet 15:353–357
4. Hunter JG, Staheli J, Oddsdottir M, Trus T (1995) Nitrous oxide pneumoperitoneum revisited. Surg Endosc 9:501–504
5. Neuman GG, Sidebotham G, Negaianu E et al (1993) Laparoscopy explosion hazards with nitrous oxide. Anesthesiology 78:875–879
6. Leighton TA (1993) Comparative cardiopulmonary effects of carbon dioxide versus helium pneumoperitoneum. Surgery 113:527–531
7. Hashizume M, Sugimachi K (1996) Trocar injury, bleeding, hernia and other complications are preventable. Fifth World Congress of Endoscopic Surgery, 13–16 March 1996, Philadelphia (SAGES handbook)
8. Nordestgaard AG, Bodily KC, Osborne Jr RW, Buttorff JD (1995) Major vascular injuries curing laparoscopic procedures. Am J Surg 169:543–545
9. Levy BS, Soderstrom RM, Dail DH (1985) Bowel injuries during laparoscopy: gross anatomy and histology. J Reprod Med 30:168
10. Hasson HM (1971) A modified instrument and method for laparoscopy. Am J Obstet Gynecol 110:886–887
11. Hurd WW, Ohl DA (1994) Blunt trocar laparoscopy. Fertil Steril 61:1177–80
12. Yuzpe AA (1990) Pneumoperitoneum needle and trocar injuries in laparoscopy: a survey on possible contributing factors and prevention. J Reprod Med 35:485–490
13. Chamberlain G, Brown JC (1978) Gynaecological laparoscopy. The report of a working party in a confidential inquiry of gynaecological laparoscopy. Royal College of Obstetricians and Gynecologists, London
14. Caprini JA, Arcelus JI, Laubach M et al (1995) Postoperative hypercoagulability and deep-vein thrombosis after laparoscopic cholecystectomy. Surg Endosc 9:304–309
15. Beebe DS, Mcnevin MP, Crain JM et al (1993) Evidence of venous stasis after abdominal insufflation for laparoscopic cholecystectomy. Surg Gynecol Obstet 176:443–447
16. Jorgensen JO, Lalak NJ, North L et al (1994) Venous stasis during laparoscopic cholecystectomy. Surg Laparosc Endosc 4:128–133
17. Millard JA, Hill BB, Cook PS et al (1993) Intermittent sequential pneumatic compression in prevention of venous stasis associated with pneumoperitoneum during laparoscopic cholecystectomy. Arch Surg 128:914–918
18. Wilson YG, Allen PE, Skidmore R, Baker AR (1994) Influence of compression stockings on lower-limb venous haemodynamics during laparoscopic cholecystectomy. Br J Surg 81:841–844
19. Ortega AE, Richman MF, Hernandez M et al (1996) Inferior vena caval blood flow and cardiac hemodynamics during carbon dioxide pneumoperitoneum. Surg Endosc 10:920–924
20. Kashtan J, Green JF, Parsons EQ, Holcroft JW (1981) Hemodynamic effects of increased abdominal pressure. J Surg Res 30:249–255

21. Marathe US, Lilly RE, Silvestry SC et al (1996) Alterations in hemodynamics and left ventricular contractility during carbon dioxide pneumoperitoneum. Surg Endosc 10:974–978
22. McLaughlin JG, Scheeres DE, Dean RJ, Bonnell BW (1995) The adverse hemodynamic effects of laparoscopic cholecystectomy. Surg Endosc 9:121–124
23. Westerband A, Van De Water JM, Amzallag M et al (1992) Cardiovascular changes during laparoscopic cholecystectomy. Surg Gynecol Obstet 175:535–538
24. Safran DB, Orlando III R (1994) Physiologic effects of pneumoperitoneum. Am J Surg 167:281–286
25. Ishizaki Y, Bandai Y, Shimomura K et al (1993) Safe intra-abdominal pressure of carbon dioxide pneumoperitoneum during laparoscopic surgery. Surgery 114:549–554
26. Philips J, Keith D, Hulka J et al (1976) Gynecologic laparoscopy in 1975. J Reprod Med 16:105–117
27. Cottin V, Delafosse B, Viale JP (1996) Gas embolism during laparoscopy. Surg Endosc 10:166–169
28. Beck DH, McQuillan PJ (1994) Fatal carbon dioxide embolism and severe haemorrhage during laparoscopic salpingectomy. Br J Anesth 72:243–245
29. Diakun TA (1991) Carbon cioxide embolism: successful resuscitation with cardiopulmonary bypass. Anesthesiology 74:1151–1153
30. Greville AC, Clements AF, Erwin DC et al (1991) Pulmonary air embolism during laparoscopic laser cholecystectomy. Anaesthesia 46:113–114
31. Ostman PL, Pantle-Fisher FH, Faure EA, Glosten B (1990) Circulatory collapse during laparoscopy. J Clin Anesth 2:129–132
32. Brantley III JC, Riley PM (1988) Cardiovascular collapse during laparoscopy: a report of two cases. Am J Obstet Gynecol 159:735–740
33. Yacoub OF, Cardona Jr I, Coveler LA, Dodson MG (1982) Carbon dioxide embolism during laparoscopy. Anesthesiology 57:533–535
34. Root B, Levy MN, Pollack S et al (1978) Gas embolism death after laparoscopy delayed by "trapping" in portal circulation Anesth Analg 57:232–237
35. Clark CC, Weeks DB, Gusdon JP (1977) Venous carbon dioxide embolism during laparoscopy. Anesth Analg 56:650–652
36. Morison DH (1974) Cardiovascular collapse in laparoscopy. Can Med Assoc J 111:433–437
37. Landercasper J, Miller GJ, Strutt PJ et al (1993) Carbon dioxide embolization and laparoscopic cholecystectomy. Surg Laparosc Endosc 3:407–410
38. Derouin M, Boudreault D, Couture P et al (1994) Detection of CO_2 venous embolism during laparosscopic surgery. Anesthesiology 81:A560
39. Durant TM, Long J, Oppenheimer MJ (1947) Pulmonary (venous) air embolism. Am Heart J 33:269–281
40. Michenfelder JD, Terry Jr HR, Daw EF, Miller RH (1966) Air embolism during neurosurgery. Anesth Analg 45:390–395
41. Wahba RWM, Tessler MJ, Kleiman SJ (1996) Acute ventilatory complications during laparoscopic upper abdominal surgery. Can J Anaesth 43:77–83
42. Dion YM, Levesque C, Doillon CJ (1995) Experimental carbon dioxide pulmonary embolization after vena cava laceration under pneumoperitoneum. Surg Endosc 9:1065–1069
43. Alvaran SB, Toung JK, Graff TE, Benson DW (1978) Venous air embolism: comparative merits of external cardiac massage, intracardiac aspiration, and left lateral decubitis position. Anesth Analg 57:166–170
44. Steffey E, Johnson BH, Eger II EI (1980) Nitrous oxide intensifies the pulmonary arterial pressure response to venous injection of carbon dioxide in the dog. Anesthesiology 52:52–55
45. Loffer FD, Pent D (1975) Indications, contraindications and complications of laparoscopy. Obstet Gynecol Surg 30:407–421
46. Prystowsky JB, Jericho BG, Epstein HM (1993) Spontaneous bilateral pneumothorax-complication of laparoscopic cholecystectomy. Surgery 114:988–992
47. Mellies CJ (1939) Pneumoperitoneum with an unusual complication. J Missouri Med Assoc 36:430–435
48. Smith CN (1943) Induced pneumoperitoneum: a fatal case. BMJ 2:404
49. Marcus DR, Lau WM, Swanstrom LL (1996) Carbon dioxide pneumothorax in laparoscopic surgery. Am J Surg 171:464–466
50. Klopfenstein CE, Gaggero G, Mamie C et al (1995) Clinical report: laparoscopic extraperitoneal inguinal hernia repair complicated by subcutaneous emphysema. Can J Anaesth 42:523–525

51. Abe H, Bandai Y, Ohtomo Y et al (1995) Extensive subcutaneous emphysema and hypercapnia during laparoscopic cholecystectomy: two case reports. Surg Laparosc Endosc 5:183–187
52. Cirocco WC, Schwartzman A, Golub RW (1994) Abdominal wall recurrence after laparoscopic colectomy for colon cancer. Surgery 116:842–846
53. Hughes ES, McDermott FT, Polglase AL, Johnson WR (1983) Tumor recurrence in the abdominal wall scar tissue after large bowel cancer surgery. Dis Colon Rectum 26:571–572
54. Boreham P (1958) Implantation metastases from cancer of the large bowel. Br J Surg 46:103–108
55. Wexner SD, Weiss EG (1996) Is laparoscopic resection for cancer safe and cost effective and equal to open resection. Fifth World Congress of Endoscopic Surgery, 13–16 March 1996, Philadelphia (SAGES handbook)
56. Fodera M, Pello MJ, Atabek U et al (1995) Trocar site tumor recurrence after laparoscopic-assisted colectomy. J Laparoendosc Surg 5:259–262
57. Fusco MA, Paluzzi MW (1993) Abdominal wall recurrence after laparoscopic-assisted colectomy for adenocarcinoma of the colon. Report of a case. Dis Colon Rectum 36:858–861
58. Whelan R, Sellers G, Allendorf J et al (1996) An in vitro model of pneumoperitoneum fails to demonstrate aerosolization of tumor cells. Fifth World Congress of Endoscopic Surgery, 13–16 March 1996, Philadelphia (in press: Surg Endosc)
59. Knolmayer TJ, Asbun HJ, Bowyer MW (1996) An experimental model of cellular aerosolization during laparoscopic surgery. Fifth World Congress of Endoscopic Surgery, 13–16 March 1996, Philadelphia (in press: Surg Endosc)
60. Hubens G, Pauwels M, Hubens A et al (1996) The influence of a pneumoperitoneum on the peritoneal implantation of free intraperitoneal colon cancer cells. Surg Endosc 10:809–812
61. Chang AE (1993) Colorectal cancer. In: Greenfield LJ, Mulholland MW, Oldham KT, Zelenock GB (eds) Surgery: scientific principles and practice. Lippincott, Philadelphia, pp 1015–1031
62. Lauroy J, Champault G, Risk N, Boutelier P (1994) Metastatic recurrence at the cannula site: should digestive carcinomas still be managed by laparoscopy? Br J Surg 81[suppl]:A31

14 Pneumoperitoneum in Cancer

J. Jakub and F.L. Greene

Introduction

The creation of pneumoperitoneum causes a host of physiologic responses which are described throughout this text. We have described in a concise manner the additional effects that must be considered when contemplating the creation of a pneumoperitoneum in a patient with cancerous disease. The use of pneumoperitoneum in a patient with cancer is unique because of the many pathophysiologic interactions that are just now beginning to be understood. The most obvious concern, and the one presently in the spotlight, is the concern of port site metastasis. In this chapter, we have attempted to summarize the important features of the relationship between pneumoperitoneum and port site recurrence, not only on a basic science level, but also from a clinical perspective.

Other issues pertaining to the cancer patient must be considered when operating laparoscopically. These include the hypercoagulable state of patients with cancer. This is important secondary to the venous stasis caused by the creation of pneumoperitoneum. Laparoscopy has many well described benefits over the traditional open approach. In addition, its preservation of the immune function becomes critical when dealing with cancer patients. This alone should lead to its continued use and further study of how it can be utilized in the patient with a cancerous disease process.

Hypercoagulability

Deep vein thrombosis (DVT) is a known complication of surgical procedures. Using radioactive fibrinogen uptake tests, Kakkar et al. [1] reported that 30% of postoperative patients developed a DVT and 10% of these patients suffered from a pulmonary embolus (PE). In a later study, Kakkar et al. [2] showed that 0.7% of patients undergoing a celiotomy, despite heparinization, experienced a pulmonary embolism.

It has been suggested that the creation of pneumoperitoneum may increase the risk of a patient developing a DVT. Virchow's triad defines venous stasis, hypercoagulability, and vascular trauma as predisposing factors for developing thromboembolism. Recent studies have documented that pneumoperitoneum induces both venous stasis and a hypercoagulable state. This, compounded with the hypercoagulable state of the cancer patient, raises legitimate concerns.

Thromboembolism as a complication of gynecological laparoscopy is rare, with a reported incidence of DVT and PE in two of 10.000 procedures [3]. With the increase in the number of laparoscopic cholecystectomies, the pathophysiological changes of pneumoperitoneum have been reassessed. Laparoscopic cholecystectomy also requires the patient to be in a reverse-Trendelenburg position for an excess of 1 h in most cases. Beebe et al. [4] showed abdominal insufflation causes venous stasis during laparoscopic cholecystectomy. Jorgensen et al. [5] confirmed this finding. They showed peak femoral blood flow velocity fell significantly and femoral vein diameter increased with the creation of pneumoperitoneum. A large increase in femoral vein blood flow was observed with the release of pneumoperitoneum. This was felt to confirm entrapment of blood within the lower limbs. This stasis is additional to any increased effect produced by the general anesthetic. A further reduction in femoral venous return would also be expected with patients in the head-up position. Decreased blood velocity with increased cross section diameter was confirmed by Ido et al. [6] in 1995 using color doppler during laparoscopic cholecystectomy. They also showed significant alterations in blood flow velocity with positional changes from supine to reverse-Trendelenburg.

Pulmonary emboli following laparoscopic cholecystectomies have been documented. It is believed that a DVT develops intraoperatively since laparoscopic cholecystectomy offers the patient a much shorter period of postoperative immobility. Jorgensen et al. [5] reported two clinically significant pulmonary emboli in his retrospective review of 487 laparoscopic cholecystectomies despite heparin therapy. Mayol et al. [7] reports a retrospective review of 200 patients with a 1% incidence of clinically significant pulmonary embolism.

Reports have indicated that open cholecystectomy activates blood coagulation. Recent results have clearly shown that laparoscopic cholecystectomy, despite being minimally invasive, also induces a significant hypercoagulable state. There is concern over whether the pneumoperitoneum itself may be responsible or at least contribute. Arginine vasopressin (AVP) is a pituitary nonpeptide whose primary physiologic role is osmoregulation. The effect of this active hormone is also known to cause constriction of the vascular bed. It has been shown that AVP is released during open cholecystectomy, and this was originally attributed to a decrease in blood pressure [8]. More recently, AVP has been shown to be released following induction of pneumoperitoneum and unrelated to changes in blood pressure. Punnonen concluded that increased intra-abdominal pressure and peritoneal distension have a direct stimulating effect on vasopressin release [9]. This increase in AVP concentration with the induction of pneumoperitoneum is important not only because of its effect on the vascular bed, but because of the role it plays in hemostasis. Nussey et al. have shown that AVP infusion causes an increase in factor VIII and von Willebrand factor (VWF). This is a dose-related phenomenon. AVP's interaction with platelets and the stimulation of factor VIII and VWF release support the hypothesis that it plays a role in the control of hemostasis, and increases the overall clotting of blood [10].

Caprini examined postoperative hypercoagulability and DVT after laparoscopic cholecystectomy and demonstrated significant postoperative hypercoagulability for the whole blood thrombelastography (TEG) index and for par-

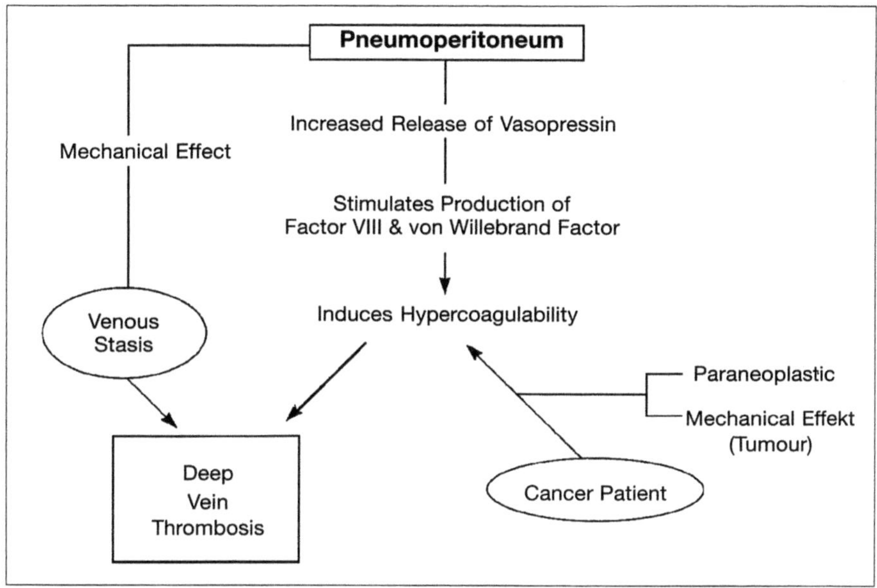

Fig. 1.   Possible effects of pneumoperitoneum and cancer patients

tial thromboplastin time (PTT). TEG has been shown to be a sensitive detector of hypercoagulability and predictor of DVT risk. They suggest that clotting activation relies more on the coagulation factors and fibrinogen than on the platelet number and function. In this study, there did not appear to be a major hemostatic response to laparotomy [11].

Because of the above findings of pneumoperitoneum's effect on venous stasis, AVP release, and possibly induction of a hypercoagulable state, the surgeon must utilize protective measures against abnormal clotting in the perioperative period. This becomes especially important in the cancer patient (Fig. 1). These effects can also be reduced by minimizing the head-up position and abdominal wall insufflation as much as possible.

Port Site Metastases

One of the greatest concerns in operating laparoscopically on patients with cancer is the fear of port site metastases. There have been numerous reports of access site metastases following a laparoscopic approach on patients with known and unknown malignancies. Reports are documented from procedures including gallbladder [12], pancreas [13], stomach [14], and colon [15], as well as lymphoma staging [16] and gynecological tumors [17]. This fear has caused many leading laparoscopists to argue that the complication may negate any theoretical advantage which may be derived using a laparoscopic approach in cancer patients. The question is whether this concern is justified.

The concept of cancer recurrence at surgical wound sites is not new. Needle track seeding of cancer following fine needle aspiration has been frequently reported. It is important to note that metastatic wound implants following open tumor resection are also documented. Hughes et al. [18], in the only study of its kind to date, prospectively followed 1603 patients who underwent curative resection for colon cancer. All of the patients with incisional recurrence died of disseminated cancer within 4 years. There were 11 cases of wound recurrence (0.7%). The first reported case following laparoscopy was in 1978 and was associated with malignant ascites [19]. Since then, with the increasing use of laparoscopy, numerous reports have surfaced and have commonly been related to an incidental finding of gallbladder cancer [20, 21]. This is not surprising since laparoscopic cholecystectomy is the most common laparoscopic procedure. More recently, however, an increased incidence of port site metastasis has followed elective laparoscopic resection for colon cancer. The concern is also heightened by the development of port site metastases at sites remote from the location of tumor extraction. In 1995, Jacobi et al. [20] reported a case in which an unsuspected gallbladder malignancy was found at the time of laparoscopic cholecystectomy. The patient was converted to an open procedure. Two months later, the patient was noted to have recurrence at two of the port sites, although the laparotomy incision was without evidence of tumor seeding. This, as well as numerous other reports, raises questions relating to the role of pneumoperitoneum and the characteristics of the trocar site in the etiology of port site recurrence [20].

The true incidence of port site metastases following laparoscopic procedures is not known at this time. The rate of access or extraction site recurrence will not be known until long-term follow-up on a large series of patients is reported. A retrospective analysis by Ramos et al. [22], which followed 208 patients undergoing laparoscopic colectomy reported an incidence of 1.44%. He argues that the majority of patients had advanced disease. He concluded that the incidence of isolated port site recurrence without diffuse peritoneal carcinomatosis was 0.48%. This study, only analyzing port extraction sites, showed recurrence with 1-year follow-up to be low. This study is obviously limited for a number of reasons:
a) only extraction sites were followed when other sites of recurrence are well documented;
b) only 83% of the surgeons surveyed responded; and
c) a short follow-up time of 1 year was reported.

Seiler [23] argues that recurrence of cancer in the standard laparotomy incision is unheard of and not mentioned in any textbooks of colorectal surgery. He reports 33 cases of port site recurrence published over a 3-year span (1993–1995) with an incidence of 6.3%. The fact that one third of the published port site recurrences are derived from patients with Duke's A and B disease is worrying and lends credence to the fact that it does not only occur in advanced disease [23].

One of the major questions regarding access site recurrence is the mode of recurrence and whether pneumoperitoneum contributes to the process. In theory, only a single cancer cell is required for malignancy to recur. Early experimental studies indicated that exfoliated cancer cells are seldom, if ever, viable as opposed to cells from other locations such as gastric cancer. This has been refuted by more recent studies which have shown a large number of viable cancer cells retrieved by in vivo colorectal lavage. Moore reported that the peritoneal lavage fluid, after surgery for malignant conditions, contained malignant cells and that this correlated with the operability of the tumor [24]. Immunocytochemical techniques were used by Juhl et al. [25], showing that 39% of patients operated upon for cancer contained intraperitoneal malignant cells. They also correlated the stage of the cancer and the presence of intraperitoneal malignancy [25]. Given that high numbers of viable tumor cells have been demonstrated, one would expect a high incidence of wound recurrence. The fact that this is not the case indicates that other factors are important.

The metastatic potential of a malignant tumor has been extensively studied. Five mechanisms of dissemination of colorectal cancer cells have been identified:
1. hematogenous,
2. lymphatic spread of circulating tumor cells,
3. exfoliated (intramural) cells in the intestinal lumen,
4. free tumor cells present in the peritoneal cavity, and
5. direct extension.

Circulating tumor cells in the blood stream were first demonstrated by Poole and Dunlop [26]. It is now clearly established that tumor cells are released into the blood stream continuously. No prognostic indicators appear to exist between this intravascular dissemination and survival [27]. Studies performed using intravenous and intra-arterial injections of tumor cells have shown these cells to implant in laparotomy wounds. However, experimental studies have shown that while intravenously injected tumor cells may implant in intraperitoneal wounds, cutaneous metastases only occur on rare occasions [28, 29]. It seems extremely unlikely in view of the recently reported incidence of intravascular tumor cells circulating in the blood stream from a colorectal source, that implantation in the lung or liver would be avoided while achieving deposition at a cutaneous site. This would mean that the malignant cell is bypassing the organs that receive all the venous drainage from the colon before the rest of the body while implanting in the abdominal wall which receives a small percent of cardiac output. The more plausible explanation is exfoliation of cells and inadvertent spillage at the time of manipulation.

Exfoliative cells in the intestinal lumen is a long established fact. Umpleby et al. [30] was able to retrieve a large number of viable cancer cells from the ends of resected colon specimens. Viable cancer cells were found proximal to the large bowel cancer in 57% of cases and distal in 84%. These cells were found at distances greater than 35 cm which supports previous reports of suture line recurrence in Duke's A and B tumors in which complete resection had been histologically confirmed. With such a high percent of viable malignant cells and a low number of recurrences, other local factors must be present to allow for growth to be established.

Jones et al. [31] have performed the only reported study thus far which examines the effect of pneumoperitoneum on access site recurrence. They injected viable human colon cancer cells into the peritoneum of hamsters and compared a control group with a group that received a 10-min pneumoperitoneum of 10 mmHg. They found trocar site implantation tripled with the addition of pneumoperitoneum (26% vs. 75%). Results of this study suggest that insufflation of the abdominal cavity with carbon dioxide(CO_2), even for a short period of time, caused enhanced tumor uptake at the laparotomy incision and trocar sites. This raises the concern that the gas pressure necessary for creating a pneumoperitoneum was sufficient to disseminate tumor cells and enhance their intraperitoneal malignant potential. In this study, both control and abdominal insufflation groups received a laparotomy incision and four trocar entrance sites. It is conceivable that increased insufflation pressures of longer duration would be expected to further increase the frequency at which tumors recur. Jones et al. [31] noted a definite dose response relationship between trocar implantation and the increasing number of cells in the inoculum. In the absence of tumor spillage, pneumoperitoneum is probably unlikely to cause tumor metastases. Their experimental tumor burden is assumed to be much higher than experienced in the clinical setting as manifest by the increased rate of laparotomy recurrence, even in the control group.

During laparoscopic colorectal surgery, the malignant tissue is dragged through a small cutaneous opening. This procedure seems to violate sound oncologic principles and is justifiably compared with Mikulicz's extra peritoneal technique. This procedure, popularized at the turn of the century, was abandoned for malignant disease following the high incidence of local recurrence resulting from exteriorizing a cancerous colon through a small incision. The local recurrence rate was 63% (15 of 24 patients) in patients who were followed for more than 4 years. Sistrunk, commenting on the operation in 1928, called it a dangerous technique and predicted that it would result in a high mortality and recurrence rate [15].

As stated above, viable exfoliative cancer cells have been documented in numerous studies, as well as metastases caused by surgical inoculation at incision sites. Inoculation by implantation of detached tumor cells on epithelial surfaces is reported in cases of spread of carcinoma from one lip to the other, from one vocal cord to the other, and from one side of the vulva to the other. Inoculation of cells can occur but is not common due to several physiological factors preventing implantation [32]. Cancer cells require adequate local factors to be present in order to survive. Past studies have shown that healing wounds may create a fertile area for cell implantation. The new capillary formation of healing wounds provides an ideal setting for tumor implantation. Murthy et al. [33] has shown experimentally that the frequency of tumor implantation is greater when cancer cells are present in wounds in their very early rather than late stages of healing [32, 33]. An immediate result of injury is hemorrhage and leakage of plasma. Upon contact with tissue pro-coagulants, plasma rapidly clots. This initial clot is a gel consisting of fibrin, fibronectin, and platelets into which inflammatory cells migrate. This forms a firm surface for which malignant cells may become adherent. Within this fibrin gel, tumor cells become trapped and shielded from the usual host defense mechanisms and, therefore, may be allowed to grow unencumbered in the abdominal wall site. It is suggested that tumor recurrence may represent selective implantation of circulating tumor cells. Though this is possible, it seems more plausible that these areas rich in potential for tumor growth would be easily inoculated by tumor cells passed through the open wound as opposed to a systemic source. In 1907, Ryall reported cancer cells on the scalpel and under the fingernails of the surgeons who did not wear gloves [34]. Malignant cells have also been known to collect on both open surgical and laparoscopic instruments [35]. It appears obvious how a metastatic lesion would develop at the site of tumor extraction. The fact that one-third of access site metastases are at port sites that were never in direct contact with the colon cancer raises significant concern that local factors are also contributory [23]. Repeated passage of instruments in and out of the port site and increased tissue handling by laparoscopic instruments may be one plausible explanation. Some have argued that there is increased tumor spillage during a laparoscopic approach secondary to decreased dexterity. Increased handling with increased exfoliation can lead to increased intraoperative spillage.

The creation of pneumoperitoneum has been indicated as a causative factor and has lead some to advocate gasless laparoscopic techniques. The creation of a pneumoperitoneum causes the peritoneal cavity to be distended at a pressure of 10–15 mmHg. This positive intraperitoneal pressure is known to have many adverse effects on cardiac, vascular, and pulmonary functions. Aside from this, there is concern that the pneumoperitoneum may have a deleterious effect on patients with intra-abdominal malignancy. The fear is that the pressure may somehow aid in metastatic spread. The methods for this include:

a) vasodilatation induced by CO_2,
b) spread of exfoliated cells by turbulent CO_2 flow into the peritoneal cavity and into and out of access ports, and
c) by directly driving malignant cells into the lymphatic and vascular systems under pressure.

During open surgery, particulate matter tends to be drawn away by the operating room ventilation system. In contrast, the pneumoperitoneum represents a closed system in which airborne particulate matter must circulate and, therefore, have an increased contact/exposure time to the abdominal organs. This may allow concentration of airborne exfoliated cells that may become trapped on the moist intraperitoneal surface. This would potentially allow these trapped cancer cells to thrive locally or be taken up and transported systemically. Although intra-abdominal manipulation of the tumor-bearing gastrointestinal tract and retroperitoneum may be a cause of dissemination of cancer cells, it has been suggested that the tumor biology of cancer cells may actually be changed by the creation of a pneumoperitoneum.

Creation of a closed operative field under pressure with insufflation of CO_2 combined with lavage aspiration would seem to favor the dissemination of micrometastases throughout the peritoneal cavity. Pneumoperitoneum promotes capillary stasis at conventional pressures of 14 mmHg. This may favor metastatic implantation of circulating cells. Tumor cells may also be spread by aerosolization. Aerosolization can occur when there is a sudden loss of pneumoperitoneum as when a laparoscopic port is inadvertently dislodged causing a sudden rush of gas through the trocar site. Similar episodes of rapid gas evacuation are seen during instrument exchange or with the deliberate venting of cautery smoke. Aerosolization can produce wide dissemination of tumor cells to essentially any part of the abdominal cavity. The return of intra-abdominal gas may also cause

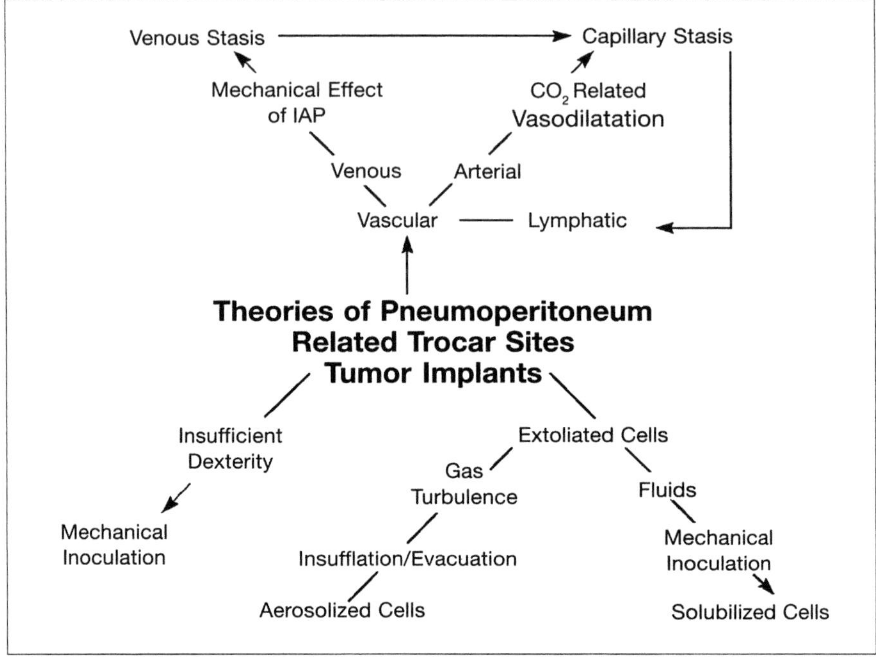

Fig. 2.   Theories of pneumoperitoneum, related trocar sites, and tumor implants

a plume with shedding of cells into the port site which could become trapped by fibrin plugs as previously described.

The true incidence of port site metastases following laparoscopic surgery is unknown at this time. Whether this phenomenon occurs more frequently following a laparoscopic approach versus the traditional open approach is also not apparent from clinical studies. Most reports of recurrences remain anecdotal and are limited to studies with short-term follow-up. The exact role played by pneumoperitoneum in the creation of metastatic disease in the cancer patient is also debatable (Fig. 2). Obviously, more information is needed to help define the role of pneumoperitoneum in the cancer patient. It must be remembered that sound oncologic principles established through scientific research cannot be jeopardized for the attainment of a new surgical approach. All of the potential benefits of minimally invasive surgery are for naught if the goal of surgical cure is not attained. At this time we do not advocate the use of laparoscopic curative resections for intra-abdominal malignancies outside of clinical trial settings.

Immunosuppression

Cancer and immunosuppression are intimately related. It is accepted that cancer patients, as a result of their disease process, are immunosuppressed. It is also an established fact that immunosuppressed patients are at much greater risk of acquiring a malignant disease. The intricacies of this relationship are just now beginning to be understood and much more research will need to be completed before we fully understand this phenomenon. Recently, minimally invasive procedures utilizing pneumoperitoneum have been evaluated for their effect on the immune system.

Injury to the host, whether it is in the form of trauma or operative intervention, has been shown on repeated occasions to suppress the immune function. This suppression of immune function is of concern in all patients because of the increased risk of infection. In the cancer patient it has been shown that surgery facilitates tumor growth in multiple studies. Surgically induced injury is associated with reproducible alterations in the host immune function and these are dependent on the severity of the injury. Therefore, the natural thought process would lead one to surmise that a minimally invasive procedure would have less effect on the immune system than an open procedure.

Laparoscopic surgery substantially reduces the extent of operative insult and will, therefore, cause less immune alterations than conventional surgery. This was demonstrated by Redmond et al. [36], comparing laparoscopic cholecystectomy with an open approach. In 1994, they demonstrated a significant increase in monocyte release of superoxide and tumor necrosis factor, neutrophil release of superoxide and chemotaxis, and white blood cell count in patients undergoing open versus laparoscopic cholecystectomy. The potential impact of decreased immunosuppression on oncological patients undergoing operative intervention is provoking.

This effect of laparotomy versus laparoscopy was investigated in 1995 by Allendorf et al. [37] on a murine model. They compared control mice (anesthesia only) to mice receiving abdominal insufflation and laparotomy. They found that:

a) laparotomy prevented the normal regression of tumors while insufflation maintained the normal pattern of tumor regression seen in controls;

b) tumors grew more aggressively after laparotomy than laparoscopy; and

c) tumors were more easily established after laparotomy than laparoscopy. This study suggests that laparotomy, but not abdominal insufflation, results in a postoperative physiologic state incapable of producing normal regression of an immunogenic tumor line. This study also suggests that laparotomy may lower the threshold number of tumor cells necessary to develop a new tumor focus, while insufflation does not [37].

The rate and incidence of tumor growth are known to be higher in immunocompromised patients. Multiple studies have demonstrated increased tumor growth after a laparotomy compared with anesthetized controls [39]. Goshima et al. [40] compared rats undergoing laparotomy versus anesthesia alone. They found a significantly greater number of pulmonary metastases after injection of tumor cells in the laparotomy cohort. They were also able to reduce tumor growth significantly on the laparotomy cohort by immunomodulation. This indicates a strong link between the immunosuppressive effects of a surgical procedure and increased tumor growth [39, 40]. Eggermont showed similar results in mice receiving intraperitoneal injection of tumor cells. Enhanced tumor growth was again established in the laparotomy group as compared to anesthetized controls [39].

To date, the study by Allendorf and coworkers is the only study comparing abdominal insufflation with laparotomy to study tumor spread. It seems logical that a laparoscopic approach would have less immunosuppressive effects than an open procedure. If it is possible to maintain oncological principles, the future will certainly have a role for minimally invasive procedures in the cancer patient.

Conclusion

With the recent widespread use of laparoscopy in the surgical field, the physiologic effects of pneumoperitoneum have become the focus of much debate and research. Central to this debate is the role pneumoperitoneum has in the cancer patient and what unique interactions need to be considered. We have attempted to focus on the three critical topics of greatest importance at this time when operating laparoscopically on a patient with cancer: hypercoagulability, immune suppression, and port site metastasis.

The cancer patient is known to be in a hypercoagulable state. Recent evidence has confirmed the effect pneumoperitoneum has on regulating the coagulation cascade. Not only is lower extremity venous stasis observed with the creation of a pneumoperitoneum, but recent studies have suggested that the body is not immune to the activation of procoagulants by minimally invasive procedures and, in fact, pneumoperitoneum may itself be the culprit. Therefore, DVT prophylaxis is of paramount importance when operating laparoscopically on these patients.

In considering the effect of pneumoperitoneum on the immune system, this interaction becomes critical when dealing with the cancer patient. Studies are beginning to show the beneficial role of laparoscopy on the immune system. Laparoscopy should offer a lowered risk for tumor growth and recurrence for patients undergoing curative resection.

Port site metastasis is presently the focus of much debate and controversy. Numerous reports of cancer recurrences at the access sites in patients with carcinomatosis as well as in patients operated on for seemingly curable disease have highlighted the concern. At this time no sound data on the incidence of port site metastasis are available. We cannot advocate the routine use of pneumoperitoneum and laparoscopy for curative resection of intra-abdominal cancer. We do feel strongly that with continued research, development of new techniques, and prospective studies, laparoscopy will have a clear role in the treatment of patients with abdominal malignancy. As discussed above, we feel that minimally invasive surgery will eventually be the modality chosen as the definitive procedure for an increasing number of malignancies.

References

1. Kakkar VV, Flang C, Howe CT, Clarke MB (1969) Natural history of postoperative deep-vein thrombosis. Lancet 2:230–232
2. Kakkar VV, Cohen AT, Edmonson RA et al (1993) Low molecular weight versus standard heparin for prevention of venous thromboembolism after major abdominal surgery. Lancet 341:259–265
3. Chamberlain G, Brown JC (1978) Gynecological laparoscopy. The report of the working party of the confidential enquiry into gynaecological laparoscopy. Royal College of Obstetricians and Gynaecologists, London
4. Beebe DS, McNevin MP, Crain JM et al (1993) Evidence of venous stasis after abdominal insufflation for laparoscopic cholecystectomy. Surg Gynecol Obstet 176:443–47
5. Jorgensen JO, Lalak NJ, North L et al (1994) Venous stasis during laparoscopic cholecystectomy. Surg Lapar Endosc 4:128–33
6. Ido K, Suzuki T, Kimura K et al (1995) Lower extremity venous stasis during laparoscopic cholecystectomy as assessed using color doppler ultrasound. Surg Endosc 9:310–313
7. Mayol J, Vincent-Hamelin E, Sarmiento JM et al (1994) Pulmonary embolism following laparoscopic cholecystectomy: report of two cases and review of the literature. Surg Endosc 8:214–217
8. Cochrane JPS, Forsling ML, Gow NM, LeQuesne LP (1981) Arginine vasopressin release following surgical operations. Br J Surg 68:209–213
9. Punnonen R, Viinamaki O (1982) Vasopressin release during laparoscopy: role of increased intra-abdominal pressure. Lancet 1:175–176
10. Nussey SS, Bevan DH, Ang VTY, Jenkins JS (1986) Effects of arginine vasopressin (AVP) infusions on circulating concentrations of platelet AVP, Factor VIII:C and von Willebrand Factor. Thromb Haemost 55:34–36
11. Caprini JA, Arcelus JI, Laubach M et al (1995) Postoperative hypercoagulability and deep-vein thrombosis after laparoscopic cholecystectomy. Surg Endosc 9:304–309
12. Barsaum GH, Windsor CW (1992) Parietal seeding of carcinoma of the gallbladder after laparoscopic cholecystectomy. Br J Surg 79:846–847
13. Siriwardena A, Samarji WN (1993) Cutaneous tumor seeding from a previously undiagnosed pancreatic carcinoma after laparoscopic cholecystectomy. Ann R Coll Surg Engl 75:199–200
14. Cava A, Roma J, Gonzales QA et al (1990) Subcutaneous metastasis following laparoscopy in gastric adenocarcinoma. Eur J Surg Oncol 16:63–67
15. Cirocco WC, Schwartzmann A, Golub RW (1994) Abdominal wall recurrence after laparoscopic colectomy for colon cancer. Surgery 116:842–846
16. Aractingi S, Marolleau JP, Daniel MT et al (1993) Localisations sous-cutane de lymphoma de Brukitt aux points de penetrations d'un coelioscope. Ann Dermatol Venereol 120:796–797
17. Hsiu JJ, Given FT, Kemp GM (1968) Tumor implantation after diagnostic laparoscopic biopsy of ovarian tumors of low malignant potential. Obstet Gynecol 68:90–93
18. Hughes ESR, McDermott FT, Polglase AL, Johnson WR (1983) Tumor recurrence in the abdominal wall scar tissue after large-bowel cancer surgery. Dis Colon Rectum 26:571–572
19. Dobronte F, Wittman T, Karlesony G (1978) Rapid development of malignant metastasis in the abdominal wall after laparoscopy. Endoscopy 10:127–130
20. Jacobi CA, Keller H, Monig S, Said S (1995) Implantable metastasis of unspected gallbladder carcinoma after laparoscopy. Surg Endosc 9:351–352
21. Copher JC, Rogers JJ, Dalton ML (1995) Trocar-site metastasis following laparoscopic cholecystectomy for unsuspected carcinoma of the gallbladder. Surg Endosc 9:348–350
22. Ramos JM, Gopta S, Anthone GJ et al (1994) Is the port-site at risk? A preliminary report. Arch Surg 129:897–900
23. Seiler CA (1995) Laparoscopic resection for colorectal cancer: a safe way to cure cancer? Digest Surg 12:302–306
24. Moore GE, Sako K, Tatsuhei K (1961) Assessment of the exfoliation of tumor cells into the body cavities. Surg Gynecol Obstet 112:469–474
25. Juhl H, Stritzel M, Wroblewski A et al (1994) Immunocytological detection of micrometastatic cells. Comparative evaluation of findings in the peritoneal cavity and the bone marrow of gastric, colorectal and pancreatic cancer patients. Int J Cancer 57:330–335

26. Pool EH, Dunlop GR (1934) Cancer cells in the bloodstream. Am J Surg 21:99–102
27. Engell HC (1959) Cancer cells in the blood: a five to nine-year follow-up study. Ann Surg 149:457–462
28. Murphy P, Alexander P, Senior PV et al (1988) Mechanisms of organ selective tumour growth by bloodborne cancer cells. Br J Cancer 57:19–31
29. Vernick J, Garside G, Hoppe E (1964) The lack of growth of intravenously inoculated tumor cells in the peripheral wounds. Cancer Res 24:1507–1508
30. Umpleby HC, Fermor B, Symes MO, Williamson RCN (1984) Viability of exfoliated colorectal carcinoma cells. Br J Surg 71:659–663
31. Jones DB, Goo LW, Reinhard MK et al (1995) Impact of pneumoperitoneum on trocar site implantation of colon cancer in hamster model. Dis Colon Rectum 38:1182–1188
32. Savalgi RS (1995) Mechanism of abdominal wall recurrence after laparoscopic resection of colonic cancers. Semin Laparosc Surg 2:158–161
33. Murthy SM, Goldschmidt RA, Rao LN et al (1989) The influence of surgical trauma on experimental metastatic cancer. Cancer 64:2036–2043
34. Ryall C (1907) Cancer infection and cancer recurrence: a danger to avoid in cancer operations. Lancet 2:1311
35. Nduka CC, Munson JRT, Mences-Gow N, Darzi A (1981) Abdominal wall metastases following laparoscopy. Br J Surg 81:648–652
36. Redmond PH, Watson WG, Houghton T et al (1994) Immune function in patients undergoing open vs laparoscopic cholecystectomy. Arch Surg 129:1240–1246
37. Allendorf JDF, Bessler M, Kayton ML et al (1995) Increased tumor establishment and growth after laparotomy vs laparoscopy in a murine model. Arch Surg 130:649–653
38. Lewis MR, Cole WH (1958) Experimental increase of lung metastases after operative trauma (amputation of limb with tumor). AMA Arch Surg 77:621–626
39. Eggermont AMM, Steller EP, Marquet RL et al (1988) Local regional promotion of tumor growth after abdominal surgery is dominant over immunotherapy with interlukin-2 and lymphokine activated killer cells. Cancer Detect Prev 12:421–429
40. Goshima H, Sagi S, Forata T et al (1989) Experimental study on preventative effects on lung metastases using LAK cells induced from various lymphocytes – special references on enhancement of lung metastasis after laparotomy stress. Jpn J Surg Soc 90:1245–1250

15 Pneumoperitoneum in the Pediatric Age

S.Z. Rubin and M.G. Davis

Introduction

A pneumoperitoneum may result from the purposeful introduction of gas into the peritoneal cavity during laparoscopy. Any transgression of the abdominal wall, however, may permit gas to enter the peritoneal cavity. Such is the case during laparotomy. Similarly, abdominal wall trauma or female genital insufflation may produce a pneumoperitoneum. Pathologically, a pneumoperitoneum may be noted following perforation of the intraperitoneal gastrointestinal tract. Bronchopulmonary air leaks may track subdiaphragmatically and produce a pneumoperitoneum. Occasionally, pneumoperitoneum is the result of gas-producing organisms.

A detailed understanding of the pathophysiology of pneumoperitoneum in childhood is required for the intelligent management of the child with a pneumoperitoneum, whether the cause be nosocomial, traumatic, or laparoscopic. The pathophysiological effect of the pneumoperitoneum itself may be inconsequential, especially when the pathological process is life-threatening, e.g., sepsis, respiratory failure. However, once the intra-abdominal volume exceeds the ability of the peritoneal cavity to expand without a significant increase in abdominal pressure, then the pneumoperitoneum per se produces serious pathophysiological sequelae. The smaller the abdominal capacity, the lower the volume threshold and the more rapid the advent of pathological effects of the pneumoperitoneum per se. Such is the case in pediatrics. If the gas present is CO_2, its absorption will result in a respiratory acidosis. The ability of the pediatric pulmonary system to compensate may be limited.

Experimental Data

Many of the studies on pneumoperitoneum and the pathologies associated with free air in the peritoneal cavities have been performed on laboratory animals (usually dogs, pigs, rats, and rabbits). The size of these animals closely equates with that of children and thus it is not surprising that the results of these studies are similar to clinical data being accumulated from the management of pediatric patients.

While pneumoperitoneum is necessary for most laparoscopic procedures, gas in the peritoneal cavity is seen in multiple pathological states. The specific pathophysiological effects of abdominal trauma, intestinal perforation, gas producing organisms, massive airway leak associated with pneumothorax, pneumo media-stinum, etc., seldom implicate the pneumoperitoneum. The main pathological process is not the presence of gas in the peritoneal cavity. If, during one of these pathological processes, the intra-abdominal pressure (IAP) increases significantly, similar pathophysiology as has been documented during experimental pneumoperitoneum may occur in addition to the effects of the primary pathology. It is doubtful whether gas in the peritoneal cavity per se induces any noticeable local effect [18]. If it is easily absorbed, it may produce systemic effects, e.g., CO_2 and respiratory acidosis [24].

Although the pathophysiological changes noted with laparoscopy are protean, laparoscopy has two major consequences, *increased IAP* and *respiratory acidosis*. The increased IAP will interfere with infradiaphragmatic venous and arterial blood flow and decrease perfusion in the intra-abdominal viscera, especially the kidney [2]. Increased IAP may restrict diaphragmatic excursion, as well as displace the diaphragm's cephalad with resultant respiratory restriction. If CO_2 is used for insufflation, then its absorption may result in changes in gas exchange or acid-base balance [13].

The ability of the abdominal cavity to accommodate increases in IAP depends on the pressure applied and the length of time during which the increased IAP is constantly present. Normal physiological transient IAP increases of up to 200 mmHg occur during coughing and defecation [2]. Peritoneal dialysis (associated with an IAP of 2–8 mmHg for the cycle) seems to produce little adverse pressure-related pathophysiology. Where IAP elevation produces ventilatory and circulatory changes, these changes are apparent within 5 min of the onset of insufflation [22]. Although IAP greater than 15 mmHg associated with a pneumoperitoneum produces significant pathophysiological effects, these effects are reversible over a 2-h period [3]. At a similar IAP without a pneumoperitoneum, no deviation from normal physiology was noted [3, 18].

Increasing IAP is effectively a 'venous tourniquet.' Blood flow from the abdomen and lower limbs is decreased while arterial perfusion persists. Central venous pressure is increased [2, 13]. This reflects the raised IAP. Cardiac output is decreased [23]. Cardiac index, left ventricular stroke work, and heart rate significantly increase [17]. The pressure on the abdominal aorta results in an elevation of blood pressure in the upper body. In young swine, when IAP is 15 mmHg, both systemic and pulmonary vascular resistance is elevated [24].

The local effects of compression of intra-abdominal arteries is most readily seen in the effect on renal function with decreased perfusion. Renal cortical blood flow is diminished at an IAP of 15 mmHg with decreased urinary output [3, 4, 19]. When the IAP exceeds 25 mmHg anuria may occur [2]. An IAP greater than 12 mmHg is associated with diminished blood flow to the liver as portal venous and superior mesenteric artery blood flow decrease, even though hepatic arterial flow is unaffected [11].

In the spontaneously ventilating animal, tidal volume and minute ventilation decrease [8]. In mechanically ventilated animals where the pressures are kept constant, the compliance of the respiratory system, the chest wall, and diaphragm decrease while the lung compliance remains constant. Dead space decreases with progressive thoracic restriction from upward diaphragmatic displacement [17].

Increased ventilation can compensate for pulmonary mechanical restriction at IAP less than 12 mmHg [18]. Both pulmonary arterial pressure and pulmonary capillary wedge pressure increase [9]. This may improve the ventilation-perfusion at IAP less than 12 mmHg and explain the lack of effect on PO_2 under these conditions.

Laparoscopy with CO_2 insufflation increases the end-tidal CO_2 in young swine with PCO_2 levels measuring up to 70 mmHg, while the pH decreases from 7.44 to 7.19, and the PO_2 showed a 37% decrease [8, 13]. These effects, particularly the changes in PO_2, are not constant and may be species specific [18, 22]. Oxygen consumption is not altered by the increased IAP and CO_2 pneumoperitoneum, indicating that the increase in PCO_2 is probably due to CO_2 absorption [14].

The effects of pneumoperitoneum are protean. Intracranial pressure (ICP) is elevated during laparoscopy with pneumoperitoneum. This elevation is additional to the presence of a raised ICP prior to the introduction of the pneumoperitoneum. In addition, the increase in ICP is independent of the changes in PCO_2 [12].

It is interesting to note that elevation of the abdominal wall as an alternative to gaseous insufflation of the abdominal cavity for the purpose of laparoscopy, which does not elevate IAP or introduce exogenous CO_2, is associated with much less noticeable elevations of central venous pressure, pulmonary arterial pressures, pulmonary capillary wedge pressures, and PCO_2 [3, 24]. Laparoscopy in 3-kg rabbits performed without increasing the intra-abdominal pressure with gas does not produce severe changes in cardiorespiratory physiology as seen when IAP is elevated with CO_2 insufflation, even when the animal is anesthetized and breathes spontaneously [15]. Alternative methods of elevating IAP, e.g., abdominal compression, did not alter pulmonary mechanics nor blood gases [18].

In summary, experimental data in adult and young animals may show similar pathophysiological effects. These effects can be classified as those due to increased intra-abdominal pressure and those due to the respiratory acidosis caused by CO_2 insufflation used for laparoscopy. Raised IAP locally decreases tissue and organ perfusion, e.g., the kidney. Circulation is profoundly affected due to raised central venous pressure, decreased cardiac output, and raised systemic arterial pressure. Elevation of the diaphragm is associated with decreased compliance and increased airway pressures. These pathophysiological changes affect homeostasis in all body tissues.

Clinical Data

Pneumoperitoneum is present during and immediately after all intraperitoneal procedures. It is a useful clinical guide in the diagnosis of the acute abdomen; but the pathophysiological effects, with the exception of air embolism, are not related to the gas in the abdomen. Thus clinical studies in this situation examine the underlying pathologies only.

The clinical use of pneumoperitoneum during laparoscopic procedures is being routinely monitored and is the subject of frequent clinical reports. More recently, the pathophysiological interaction between anesthesia and the raised IAP from CO_2 insufflation, is the subject of clinical investigation.

Raised Intra-abdominal Pressure

The clinical observations are very similar to those seen in laboratory animals. Essentially, the effect is related to the level of IAP, its duration, and the size of the animal. Clinically, cardiopulmonary insufficiency has been observed in children resulting from a raised IAP secondary to ascites, enlarging retroperitoneal tumors, visceromegaly, peritonitis, etc. Limited elevation of IAP may clinically produce little obvious effect. For example, during routine peritoneal dialysis where measured pressures range from 2–8 mmHg, there are no adverse pressure-related effects. However, the clinician must be aware of the possible presentation or exacerbation of abdominal wall hernial defects and gastroesophageal reflux when IAP is elevated [2].

Hsing et al. noted that there were no observed hemodynamic effects of a 10-mmHg IAP present for 15 min in infants and children ranging in age from 11 months to 13 years [10]. During CO_2 insufflation with an IAP of 12 mmHg, peak inspiratory airway pressures increased by greater than 40% and compliance of the respiratory system decreased by 47%; there was no increase in dead space [14]. Following release of the pneumoperitoneum, the respiratory mechanics remained abnormal [1]. The smaller the child, the more rapid the observed increase in pneumoperitoneum-associated airway pressures. In this study, where the IAP was maintained at 10 mmHg, there was no effect on O_2 saturation [10].

In the presence of preexisting decreased cardiac output, e.g., congenital heart disease, sepsis, the decreased venous return, increased heart rate, and raised systemic arterial blood pressure resulting from the increased abdominal pressure may result in acute cardiac failure, especially in small infants. Restriction of intravenous fluids during laparoscopy may not influence the cardiovascular pathophysiology.

Carbon Dioxide Insufflation

The expected increase in end tidal $ETCO_2$ was noted in all pediatric age groups [10]. As in animals, the expected increase in PCO_2 and fall in pH was noted following intraperitoneal insufflation of CO_2. This reflected absorption across the peritoneal membrane. To correct these absorbed abnormalities, minute ventilation needs to be increased to maintain normal blood gases. Intra-operative increase in tidal volume and respiratory rate may be necessary to maintain normal blood gases. Postoperative expiratory PCO_2 remained elevated for up to 3 h, reflecting retained intraperitoneal CO_2 and tissue CO_2 stores. The use of narcotics which suppress respiration will exacerbate this effect [21]. Notwithstanding the above, postoperative pulmonary function tests, blood gases, narcotic use, and length of hospitalization all favored laparoscopy in a clinical comparison of laparotomy and laparoscopy for nephrectomy [5].

Of importance is the clinical observation that extra-peritoneal CO_2 produces a greater and quicker elevation in PCO_2, suggesting that the absorption of CO_2 from the loose connective tissues is enhanced when compared to CO_2 absorption from the peritoneal cavity [16, 25].

Laparoscopy and Anesthesia

The physiologic effects of anesthesia, muscle relaxation, narcotics, and positive pressure ventilation interact with the pathophysiological changes caused by a positive pressure CO_2 pneumoperitoneum. Respiratory physiology is affected early. Although adults may tolerate brief (less than 30 min) laparoscopic procedures while spontaneously ventilating [7], the smaller the patient the faster and more pronounced the increase in respiratory pressures and mechanical restriction. The rapid absorption of CO_2 causes even further elevation of the PCO_2. Thus in children it is probably safer when using CO_2 insufflation to use muscle paralysis and controlled ventilation. Minute ventilation should be increased to maintain normal respiratory function and blood gases.

Postoperative prolonged elevations of expiratory CO_2 may continue for more than 3 h. The administration of narcotics suppresses the CO_2 effect on ventilation and may result in hypoventilation with further CO_2 retention [21].

The clinical effects of raised IAP are protean; as more systems are monitored further pathophysiology is documented. The increase in cerebral blood flow seen may be due to PCO_2 elevation [6].

The diagnosis of technical complications such as pneumothorax, air embolism, extraperitoneal insufflation of CO_2, and vascular and intestinal injuries is essential, but the pathophysiology of these complications in combination with the pneumoperitoneum have not been studied.

Conclusions

The presence of a pneumoperitoneum is an important clinical diagnostic sign in acute abdominal and thoracic emergencies. The pathophysiological effects of the pneumoperitoneum in these conditions have not been studied. Since laparoscopy is increasingly being used in the treatment of these diseases it will be important to document and understand the effects of the pneumoperitoneum since they may effect the management of the patient.

The infant is primarily a diaphragmatic breather. Increased IAP restricts the excursion of the diaphragm. Furthermore, the insufflation of CO_2 into the peritoneal cavity of a child (or small animal), may result in rapid diffusion of CO_2 into the bloodstream with a catastrophic effect on gas exchange.

Correction of these abnormalities has been achieved by increasing the minute ventilation [20] or by altering the balance of pressures across the diaphragm by placing the animal in the Trendelenburg position [23]. Although these effects in the ventilated, paralyzed normal infant may be minimal [18], laparoscopy in the sick infant with compromised respiratory function may result in circulatory and/ or respiratory insufficiency.

The respiratory effects of increased IAP and intraperitoneal CO_2 require careful monitoring of respiratory mechanics, including airway pressures, tidal volume, respiratory rate (minute ventilation), pulmonary compliance, in addition to blood gases, pH, and $ETCO_2$ [1]. The smaller the patient, the more critical the monitoring.

The pathophysiological changes associated with raised IAP and CO_2 insufflation need to be carefully evaluated in the child with compromised cardiopulmonary function. Increased IAP may cause inferior vena caval (IVC) compression and a rise in arterial blood pressure. The heart rate increases probably as a response to decreased ventricular stroke volume and cardiac output. Raised IAP affects all the abdominal viscera. While the pressure on the kidney will directly result in decreased urinary output; the liver will be underperfused. It would appear that as long as the IAP is kept below 12 mmHg these pathophysiological changes are easily managed [17].

Anesthesia itself may result in hypoventilation, acidosis, atelectasis, and decreased cardiac output, etc. Controlled volume ventilation with modification of the minute volume is prudent [20]. Cautious use of narcotics which depress respiration and medications which suppress cardiac function and circulatory homeostatic mechanisms is advised. Continuous assessment of cardiovascular, respiratory, and renal functions is essential during laparoscopic procedures and in the immediate 3-h postoperative period. The anesthetist must be aware of the danger of regurgitation due to the exacerbation of gastroesophageal reflux as a consequence of raised IAP [2].

In children, the size of the abdomen restricts the volume of gas it can contain. Even a small amount of insufflated gas may exceed the elastic limit of stretch of the small abdominal cavity. The pathophysiological changes in the respiratory and circulatory systems appear more rapidly the smaller the child. The difficulty of maintaining a sufficient pneumoperitoneum for the performance of the technical procedure may be difficult, especially when the change of the instruments at the ports will be associated with significant loss of insufflated gas. Thus the procedure may be longer in children. The already compromised "therapeutic window" for safe laparoscopy in the small child is further contracted by the presence of any disease process which affects circulatory or respiratory function, e.g., congenital heart disease, sepsis, anemia. Large flows of cold CO_2 may produce hypothermia further depressing cardiopulmonary function [17]. The use of the standard CO_2 insufflation laparoscopy in such patients must be carefully considered. The smaller and sicker the infant, the greater the contraindication for laparoscopy with CO_2 insufflation. Anesthesia for pediatric laparoscopy requires special vigilance and adequate monitoring. IAP should not exceed 12 mmHg.

Summary

The pathophysiology of pneumoperitoneum is summarized in Figure 1. If our goal is to apply the less invasive technique of laparoscopic surgery to a wider group of children, then special care should be taken in the following clinical situations:

1. *Neonates and infants.* These patients have small physiological volumes and will show the effects of raised IAP with CO_2 insufflation more rapidly and at lower pressures. The use of the present standard laparoscopic techniques in small infants with compromised respiratory and cardiovascular systems, e.g., congenital heart disease, sepsis, respiratory distress, requires special caution.

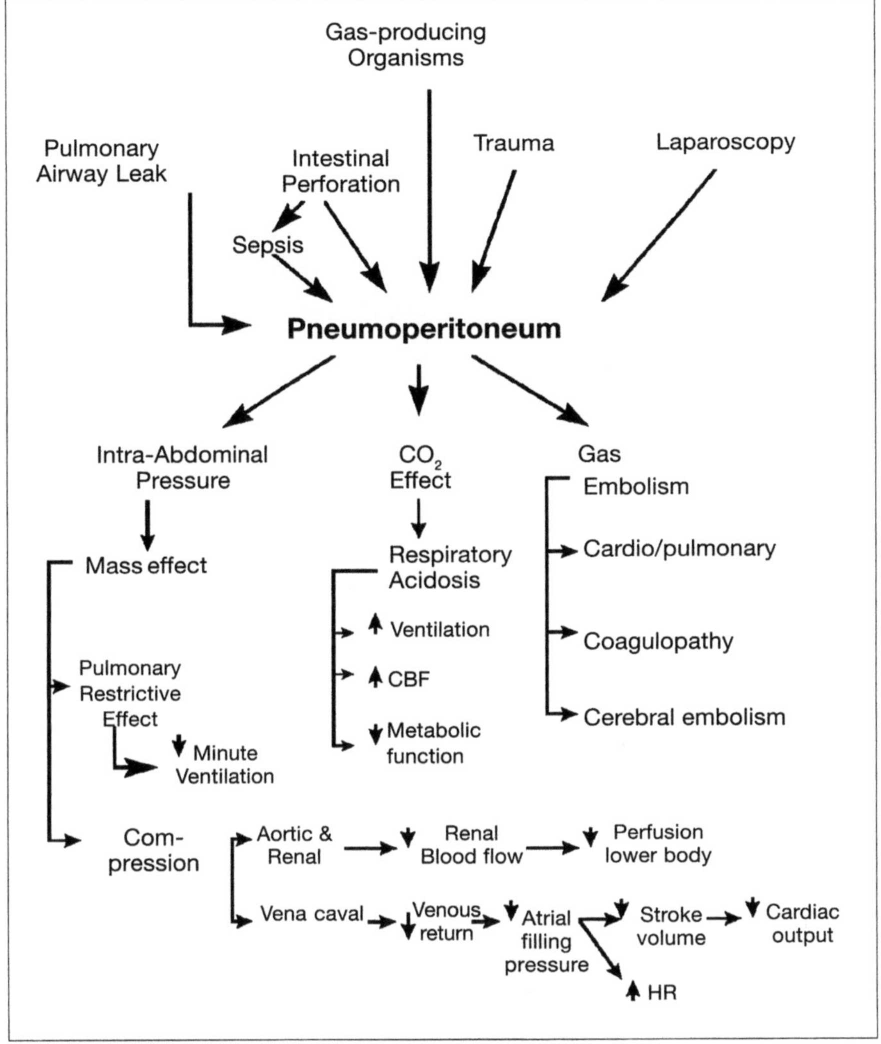

Fig. 1.   Pathophysiology of pneumoperitoneum. *CBF*, cerebral blood flow; *HR*, heart rate

2. *Multiple trauma.* The depression in cardiac output, the potential for acidosis, the decreased renal perfusion, and the raised ICP with increased cerebral blood flow which are associated with the elective use of laparoscopy with raised IAP and CO₂ insufflation, all indicate extra care if laparoscopy is to be used in a situation where all these systems may be compromised prior to the commencement of surgery.

It is possible that children falling into this patient category would benefit from the refinement of new laparoscopic techniques which do not require raised IAP and CO_2 insufflation.

References

1. Bardoczky GI, Engelman E, Levarlet M, Simon P (1993) Ventilatory effects of pneumoperitoneum monitored with continuous spirometry. Anaesthesia 48:309–11
2. Carry PY, Banssillon V (1994) La pression intra-abdominale. Ann Fr Anesth Reanim 13:381–99
3. Chiu AW, Chang LS, Birkett DH, Babayan RK (1995) The impact of pneumoperitoneum, pneumo-retroperitoneum, and gasless laparoscopy on the systemic and renal hemodynamics. J Am Coll Surg 181:397–406
4. Chiu AW, Azadzoi KM, Hatzichristou DG, Siroky MB, Krane RJ, Babayan RK (1994) Effects of intra-abdominal pressure on renal tissue perfusion during laparoscopy. J Endo Urol 8:99–103
5. Eden CG, Haigh AC, Carter PG, Coptcoat MJ (1994) Laparoscopic nephrectomy results in better post-operative pulmonary function. J Endo Urol 8:419–423
6. Fujii Y, Tanaka H, Tsuruoka S, Toyooka H, Amaha K (1994) Middle cerebral arterial blood flow velocity increases during laparoscopic cholecystectomy. Anesth Analg 78:80–83
7. Goodwin AP, Rowe WL, Ogg TW (1992) Day case laparoscopy. A comparison of two anaesthetic techniques using the laryngeal mask during spontaneous breathing. Anaesthesia 47:892–895
8. Gross ME, Jones BD, Bergstresser DR, Rosenbauer RR (1993) Effects of abdominal insufflation with nitrous oxide on cardiorespiratory measurements in spontaneously breathing isoflurane-anesthetized dogs. Am J Vet Res 54:1352–1358
9. Ho HS, Gunther RA, Wolfe BM (1992) Intraperitoneal carbon dioxide insufflation and cardiopulmonary functions. Laparoscopic cholecystectomy in pigs. Arch Surg 127:928–933
10. Hsing CH, Hseu SS, Tsai SK, Chu CC, Chen TW, Wei CF, Lee TY (1995) The physiological effect of CO_2 pneumoperitoneum in pediatric laparoscopy. Acta Anaesthesiol Sin 33:1–6
11. Ishizaki Y, Bandai Y, Shimomura K, Abe H, Ohtomo Y, Idezuki Y (1993) Safe intra-abdominal pressure of carbon dioxide pneumoperitoneum during laparoscopic surgery. Surgery 114:549–554
12. Josephs LG, Este-McDonald JR, Birkett DH, Hirsch EF (1994) Diagnostic laparoscopy increases intracranial pressure. J Trauma 36:815–819
13. Liem T, Applebaum H, Herzberger B (1994) Hemodynamic and ventilatory effects of abdominal CO_2 insufflation at various pressures in the young swine. J Pediatr Surg 29:966–969
14. Luiz T, Huber T, Hartung HJ (1992) Veranderungen der Ventilation wahrend laparoskopischer Cholezystektomie. Anaesthetist 41:520–526
15. Luks FI, Peers KH, Deprest JA, Lerut TE (1995) Gasless laparoscopy in infants: the rabbit model. J Pediatr Surg 30:1206–1208
16. Mullett CE, Viale JP, Sagnard PE, Miellet CC, Ruynat LG, Counioux HC, Motin JP, Boulez JP, Dargent DM, Annat GJ (1993) Pulmonary CO_2 elimination during surgical procedures using intra- or extraperitoneal CO_2 insufflation. Anesth Analg 76:622–626
17. Rayman R, Girotti M, Armstrong K, Inman KJ, Lee R, Girvan D (1995) Assessing the safety of pediatric laparoscopic surgery. Surg Laparosc Endosc 5:437–443
18. Rubin SZ, Davis GM, Sehgal Y, Kaminski MJ (1996) Does laparoscopy adversely affect gas exchange and pulmonary mechanics in the newborn? An experimental study. J Laparoendosc Surg 6:69–73
19. Shuto K, Kitano S, Yoshida T, Bandoh T, Mitarai Y, Kobayashi M (1995) Hemodynamic and arterial blood gas changes during carbon dioxide and helium pneumoperitoneum in pigs. Surg Endosc 9:1173–1178
20. Tan PL, Lee TL, Tweed WA (1992) Carbon dioxide absorption and gas exchange during pelvic laparoscopy. Can J Anaesth 39:677–681
21. Tolksdorf W, Strang CM, Schippers E, Simon HB, Truong S (1992) Die Auswirkungen des Kohlendioxid-Pneumoperitoneums zur laparoskopischen Cholezystektomie auf die postoperative Spontanatmung. Anaesthetist 41:199–203
22. Windberger U, Siegl H, Woisetschlager R, Schrenk P, Podesser B, Losert U (1994) Hemodynamic changes during prolonged laparoscopic surgery. Eur Surg Res 26:1–9

23. Williams MD, Murr PC (1993) Laparoscopic insufflation of the abdomen depresses cardiopulmonary function. Surg Endosc 7:12–6
24. Woolley DS, Puglisi RN, Bilgrami S, Quinn JV, Slotman GJ (1995) Comparison of the hemodynamic effects of gasless abdominal distention and CO_2 pneumoperitoneum during incremental positive end-expiratory pressure. J Surg Res 58:75–80
25. Wurst H, Finsterer U (1994) Emphysem bei laparoskopischer Chirurgie. Veranderungen der pulmonalen CO_2-Elimination. Anaesthetist 43:466–468

16 Laparoscopic Surgery in Pregnancy

J.K. Silva and L.D. Platt

Introduction

Surgical emergencies requiring abdominal exploration are uncommon during pregnancy. The estimated frequency of nonobstetric surgery during pregnancy is approximately 0.75%–2% [4]. The most common nonobstetric/nongynecologic condition requiring surgical treatment in the pregnant patient is acute appendicitis, followed by acute cholecystitis [21]. With the exception of ectopic pregnancy, laparotomy remains the current gold standard for intra-abdominal surgery in the obstetric population. In the nonobstetric population, however, laparoscopy has become the most popular method. The benefits of laparoscopy include: shorter operating time, and thereby less exposure to anesthetic agents [8], the ability to diagnose and treat during the same procedure [19], less postoperative pain, minimization of postoperative pulmonary complications [15], rapid return of gastrointestinal function, and smaller incisions, all resulting in shorter hospital stays and faster recoveries [14, 16]. These benefits are equally relevant to the obstetric population; however, data regarding the safety of laparoscopy [4] and the effects of prolonged carbon dioxide pneumoperitoneum on the fetus are sparse [20]. Pregnancy, therefore, remains a relative contraindication to laparoscopy [20], despite case reports attesting to its safety and favorable perinatal outcome [18, 19, 21]. As surgeons gain expertise in laparoscopic procedures, one can foresee a concomitant increase in the performance of laparoscopy in the pregnant patient [4]. It is prudent, therefore, to familiarize ourselves with the principles of laparoscopically induced pneumoperitoneum and anticipate the pathophysiologic effects it may have on the mother and fetus.

Pneumoperitoneum in Pregnancy

Three basic but important concerns arise when dealing with the pregnant patient undergoing laparoscopic surgery:
1. The maternal physiologic alterations associated with pregnancy;
2. factors unique to pregnancy and pneumoperitoneum that can affect utero-placental blood flow; and
3. the overall effect of these influences on the well-being of the fetus.

Maternal Physiology

Physiologic adaptations in pregnancy occur early in the first trimester and continue throughout gestation. Hormonal changes in the first trimester, mechanical effects of the gravid uterus in the second trimester, and the increasing metabolic demand throughout pregnancy affect all organ systems [4]. The systems that are uniquely affected by pneumoperitoneum, and therefore important to address in the preparation of the gravida for laparoscopic surgery will be discussed.

Cardiovascular System

Cardiac output starts to increase as early as 5 weeks after the last menstrual period, reaching a level of approximately 50% above the nonpregnant state by the end of the second trimester [4]. Mean arterial blood pressure falls in mid-gestation and returns to prepregnant levels at term [4]. In studies involving pregnant ewes, maternal perfusion pressure decreased approximately 22% in response to peritoneal insufflation with carbon dioxide to 20 mmHg, resulting in a 61% reduction in placental blood flow compared to matched controls. While this did not appear to have any effect on fetal perfusion pressure, blood flow, pH, or blood gas tensions, more studies are needed before one can extrapolate these findings to humans [2]. Extrapolating from human studies in the nonpregnant population, it seems likely that intra-abdominal pressures above 20 mmHg may reduce cardiac output and blood pressure sufficiently to result in some decrease in uteroplacental blood flow [4]. The extent to which this affects the fetus awaits further investigation.

On the other hand, it is well known that the weight of the uterus in the second half of gestation compresses the inferior vena cava in the supine position resulting in hypotension and a reduction in cardiac output of 25%–30% [4]. This alone can compromise uterine and fetal blood flow which can be worsened by the additional decrease in cardiac output created by pneumoperitoneum.

Respiratory System

Alveolar ventilation increases by 25% by the 16th week of gestation to a maximum of 70% at term, thereby resulting in a chronic respiratory alkalosis and a *PaCO$_2$ level of approximately 30 mmHg. During general anesthesia it is important to control minute ventilation to maintain this lower PaCO$_2$ level because normal levels associated with nonpregnant women will result in acute respiratory acidosis [5]. Functional residual capacity is reduced by 20% [4, 5], resulting in increased alveolar dead space and decreased oxygen reserve [4, 17]. This may be further exacerbated by the decrease in functional residual capacity created by pneumoperitoneum.

Renal System

Effective renal plasma flow and glomerular filtration rate are both increased as pregnancy advances. Urine output does not reflect this increase and changes little if at all throughout pregnancy [11]. There does appear, however, to be a positional effect in that effective renal plasma flow, glomerular filtration rate, and urinary output are all reduced in the supine and upright position [11]. The decrease in urinary output created by pneumoperitoneum may lead to further reduction in urinary output than might be seen in the nonobstetric population, particularly in the head-up position employed in laparoscopic cholecystectomy. Release of vasopressin in response to decreased blood pressure resulting from intra-abdominal pressures above 20 mmHg may be another factor contributing to low urine output [6].

Gastrointestinal System

As pregnancy progresses the stomach is displaced from its normal vertical position, with subsequent displacement of the intra-abdominal portion of the esophagus into the thorax. This results in a reduction in lower esophageal sphincter tone and places the pregnant woman at increased risk for aspiration. This also prevents the normal rise in lower esophageal sphincter tone that accompanies increases in intragastric pressure [5]. The risk of gastric aspiration is therefore likely to be greater in the pregnant patient undergoing laparoscopic surgery due to the increase in intra-abdominal pressure created by pneumoperitoneum. Any patient beyond 18 weeks of gestation should be considered at high risk for gastric aspiration due to the mechanically induced factors created by increasing uterine growth [5].

Vascular System

Pregnancy is a hypercoagulable state. The venous stasis created by the increased intra-abdominal pressure from pneumoperitoneum, as well as positioning in surgery, place the pregnant patient at substantial risk for deep venous thrombosis. Preventive measures such as graded compression stockings or intermittent sequential pneumatic compression with or without subcutaneous heparin should be initiated at the onset of surgery to minimize this risk.

Uteroplacental Blood Flow

Uterine blood flow increases throughout pregnancy, reaching a maximum of approximately 600–700 cc/min at term. The distribution of the cardiac output to the uterus also increases. Blood flow to the uterus will therefore decrease whenever perfusion pressure decreases or uterine vascular resistance increases [6]. Decreases in blood pressure either by caval compression due to supine positioning, and/or increased intra-abdominal pressure, will not only decrease uterine perfusion, but will also increase uterine vascular resistance by way of the renin–angiotensin pathway activated to help maintain systemic blood pressure [6]. Both of these mechanisms act synergistically to maintain systemic blood pressure at the expense of uterine blood flow, thereby placing the fetus at risk of hypoxia and acidosis.

Fetal Adaptations

Organogenesis is almost complete by 56 days postfertilization [10]. While major insults to the embryo prior to 17 days postfertilization usually have an "all or nothing effect," days 17–56 are the most vulnerable for the embryo [10]. After day 60, there is little susceptibility to structural congenital malformation. The remainder of the gestation period is characterized by organ growth and central nervous system development. Any insult during this time period is therefore likely to result in both growth and central nervous system developmental dysfunction [10].

Fetal oxygenation depends on maternal oxygenation. Mild to moderate decreases in maternal PaO_2 is well tolerated by the fetus because of the high concentration of fetal hemoglobin present which has a high affinity for oxygen [4]. Aside from this, the fetus has almost no oxygen reservoir and must rely on continuous maternal transplacental oxygen transfer [9], making it vulnerable to asphyxia in the presence of maternal hypotension of any cause [4]. Maternal hyperventilation or other factors resulting in alkalosis can also compromise maternal-fetal oxygen transfer by umbilical artery constriction, causing increased uteroplacental blood flow resistance [3], and by shifting the maternal oxyhemoglobin curve to the left [4]. Because of the large maternal–fetal oxygen tension gradient, fetal PaO_2 never exceeds 60 mmHg, despite increases in maternal PaO_2. Fetal $PaCO_2$, however, correlates directly with maternal levels which in the face of maternal hypercapnia, can result in fetal acidosis, myocardial depression, and hypotension [4].

Compromise in fetal oxygenation can be seen in the fetal heart rate tracing, particularly after 25 weeks gestation when heart rate variability, a good indicator of fetal well-being, is present [7]. One must be aware that drugs, particularly opioids and anesthetic induction agents, can decrease fetal heart rate variability [7]. Persistent bradycardia in the absence of variability, however, is an ominous sign reflecting fetal distress [4]. In the event of persistent fetal bradycardia, resuscitative measures must be initiated promptly. Hemostasis should be secured and confirmed, and maternal positioning, oxygenation, and hydration optimized simultaneously. If the fetus does not respond favorably with a correction in the heart tracing within 5 min, and the fetus is of at least 25 weeks gestation, preparation for emergent cesarean delivery must be initiated to optimize fetal outcome.

Precautions in Pregnancy

Most studies on intra-abdominal surgery in pregnancy site major complications affecting fetal well-being as being related to operative delay and disease severity at the time of diagnosis rather than the surgical procedure itself [1, 4]. The decision to perform laparoscopy must therefore be clearly made based on sound criteria and judgment and guided by the potential benefit of such procedure in comparison to the standard laparotomy approach. Any operative procedure in pregnancy must be clearly indicated; as such, laparoscopy, however brief, must never be performed on an elective basis.

Time and Exposure

The duration of any surgical procedure in pregnancy should be limited to minimize the inherent risk of prolonged anesthesia on the fetus. Laparoscopy is no exception. If the experience of the surgeon is such that the procedure might take longer lapaorscopically, it might be best to refer to a surgeon with more experience, or perform the operation via laparotomy.

Gestational Age

Accurate dating of the pregnancy preoperatively is important, not only to determine or confirm gestational age, but also to obtain baseline biometry against which postoperative growth of the fetus can be compared.

The second trimester is the optimal time to operate as it avoids the period of organogenesis associated with the first trimester, and the susceptibility to induce premature labor and delivery in the third trimester. Surgical procedures that do not involve uterine manipulation incur the lowest risk of preterm labor [4]. It is therefore prudent to evaluate uterine size and feasibility of the laparoscopic approach in providing adequate visibility of abdominal organs without undue uterine manipulation. With advancing gestation, the uterus is also at greater risk of injury; however, because there is no consensus on the gestational age at which the uterus will limit lapaoroscopic access [21], each case must be assessed individually and matched with the operator's expertise and level of comfort.

Positioning

Care must be taken in both the Trendelenburg and head-up positions to position the mother on her left side to avoid supine hypotension, compromise of uterine blood flow, and fetal hypoxia.

Risk of Thromboembolism

The hypercoagulable state of pregnancy and venous stasis incurred with surgery places the pregnant patient at substantial risk of deep venous thrombosis and its sequelae. Graded compression stockings or intermittent pneumatic compression with or without prophylactic subcutaneous heparin at the onset of surgery should be standard protocol.

Maternal Ventilation

Care must be taken to minimize the development of hypercarbia. To this end, carefully controlled mechanical ventilation should be employed to keep maternal $PaCO_2$ near the 30-mmHg norm for pregnancy. Intra-abdominal pressures should also be limited to 12–15 mmHg and, if feasible, the lowest pressure possible to allow adequate visualization of organs and safe manipulation of surgical instruments. If this cannot be accomplished with intra-abdominal pressures below 15 mmHg, laparotomy may be best in order to prevent serious hemodynamic compromise associated with higher pressures.

Urine Output

The effect of pneumoperitoneum on urine output, although reversible, requires adequate hydration preoperatively, and careful surveillance intraoperatively to optimize renal blood flow. As with any nonobstetric patient, this monitoring should extend into the postoperative period to assure adequate return of function.

Risk of Aspiration

Pregnancy places the patient at increased risk of gastric aspiration. Precautions must therefore be taken to minimize gastric acidity preoperatively. Liberal use of a nasogastric tube to assure gastric emptying and careful patient positioning intraoperatively are additional measures used to minimize risk.

Fetal Monitoring

Documentation of fetal life by auscultation and/or continuous tracing is essential prior to surgery. Intraoperative intermittent auscultation of the fetal heart rate is feasible from 18 weeks gestation; however, continuous monitoring would not be indicated until actual fetal viability, which occurs at approximately 25 weeks gestation, and prior to this time, may be technically difficult [4].

The development of the laparoscopic Doppler probe, traditionally used to locate intra-abdominal vessels, particularly in laparoscopic varicocele ligation [12, 13], can be a useful tool to evaluate the fetal heart rate intraoperatively. This semiflexible probe can fit through a 5-mm port, is easily maneuvered [12, 13], and connects to a speaker that can be placed on or off the operative field [13],

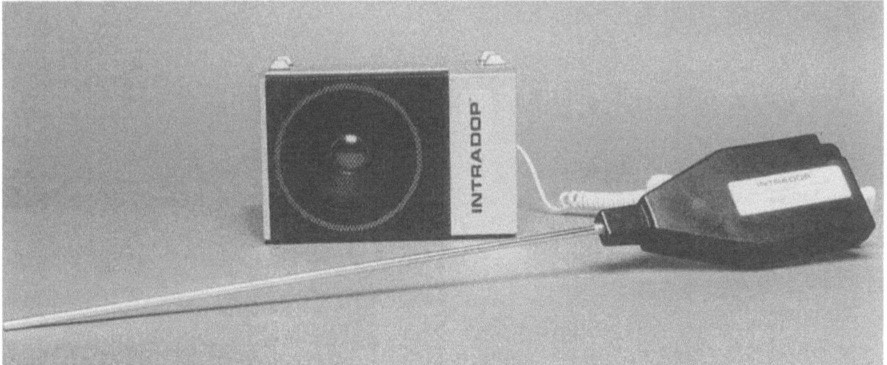

Fig. 1. Laparoscopic Doppler probe

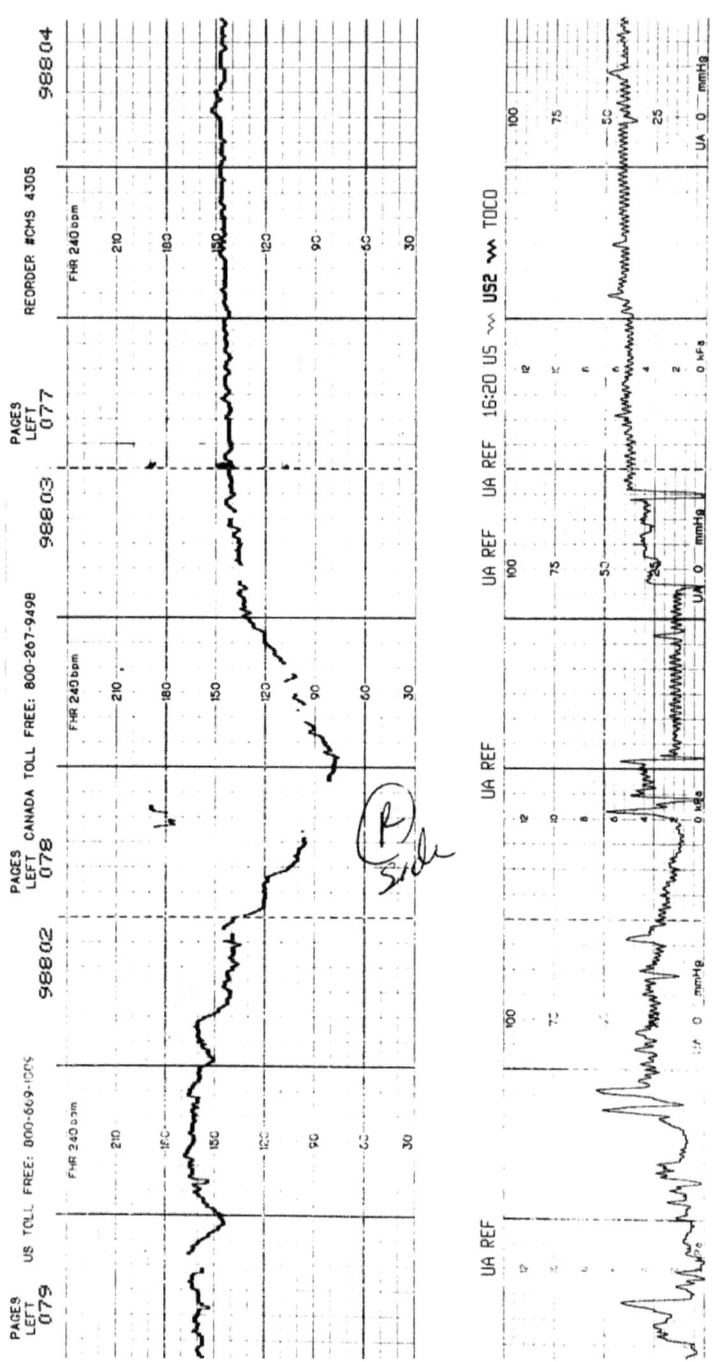

Fig. 2a

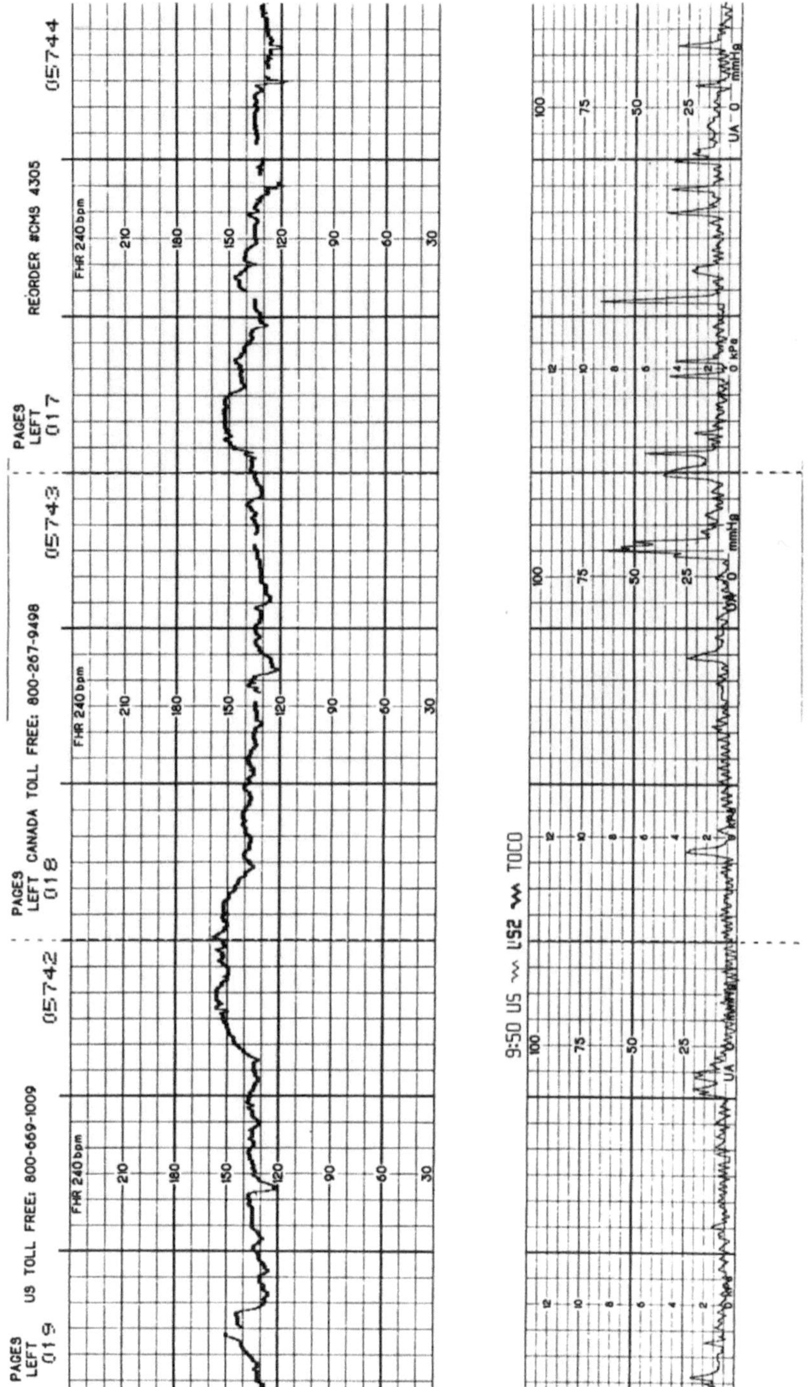

Fig. 2b

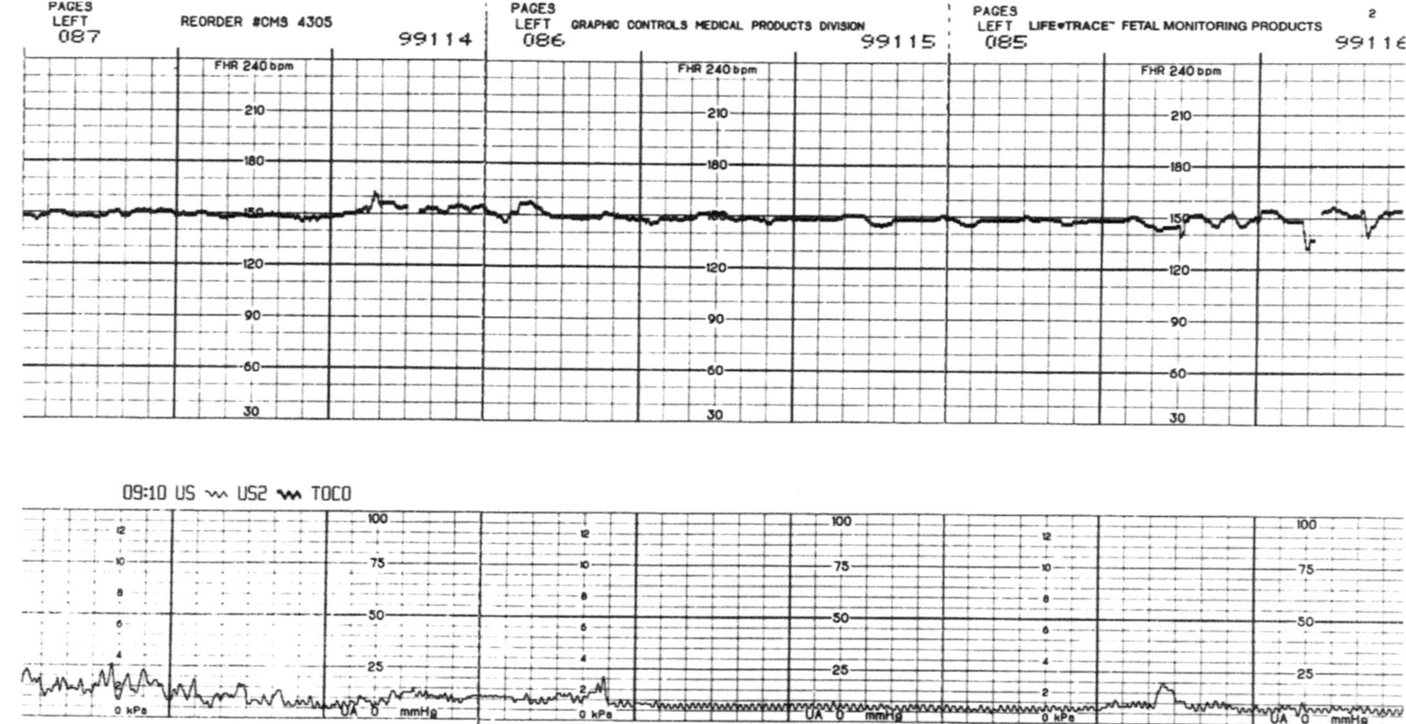

Fig. 2a-c.   **a** Prolonged bradycardia in a fetus confirmed by the laparoscopic Doppler probe. **b** Fetal heart tracing with good variability. **c** Fetal heart tracing with decreased variability thereby allowing fetal heart rate auscultation without any undue risk of violating sterile technique as can occur with intra-operative external monitoring (Fig. 1). This method can easily confirm fetal life and abrupt alterations in the fetal heart rate, in particular, prolonged bradycardia (Fig. 2a). However, this method does not produce a continuous visual fetal heart rate tracing, and is therefore unable to portray fetal heart rate variability or other subtle alterations and trends (Fig. 2b, c).

The decision to intervene for fetal compromise detected intraoperatively should be made beforehand, and preparation for abdominal delivery and subsequent resuscitation in place prior to the onset of surgery. Fortunately, the fetus is a good indicator of maternal volume and acid–base status. Therefore, acute changes in the heart tracing should alert the surgeon to carefully assess the maternal position, blood pressure, oxygenation, acid–base status, and surgical site and correct any perturbations before proceeding with emergent delivery.

Fetal monitoring postoperatively is also important for the viable fetus with intervention for fetal distress undertaken only after correctable maternal causes have been ruled out, or intervention for such proven unsuccessful. If the fetal tracing is nonreactive, a biophysical profile is indicated to assess amniotic fluid, fetal breathing, movement, and tone as indicators of fetal well-being.

Uterine Activity

Minimization of uterine manipulation appears to be the most important factor affecting uterine activity in the postoperative period [4]. In a 17-year prospective study on pregnant patients undergoing laparotomy, Allen et al. (1989) determined the risk to the fetus of preterm labor to be approximately 15%–20% [1]. The use of liberal tocolysis in these patients proved helpful (Allen et al. 1989); however, the prophylactic use of tocolysis is not without risk and remains controversial [4]. A baseline preoperative cervical examination with reservation of tocolysis for those at risk of preterm labor (i.e., history of preterm labor), significant perioperative uterine activity, and/or documented cervical change, is probably best.

Summary (See figures 3 and 4)

The frequency of laparoscopic surgery for nonobstetric indications during pregnancy is likely to increase in the near future. While many benefits can be cited for this approach, the pathophysiologic effects of pneumoperitoneum on the mother and fetus dictate that gravid candidates be carefully selected, and that the operation be performed by surgeons with expertise in the technique to avoid unnecessarily lengthy procedures with excessive uterine manipulation. Indications for laparoscopic surgery in pregnancy include ectopic pregnancy, ovarian torsion, acute appendicitis, acute cholecystitis, and undiagnosed acute abdomen. If nonemergent, as in cases involving nonacute abdominal or pelvic masses, laparoscopy should ideally be limited to the second trimester so as to avoid interference with organogenesis, and minimize susceptibility to premature labor

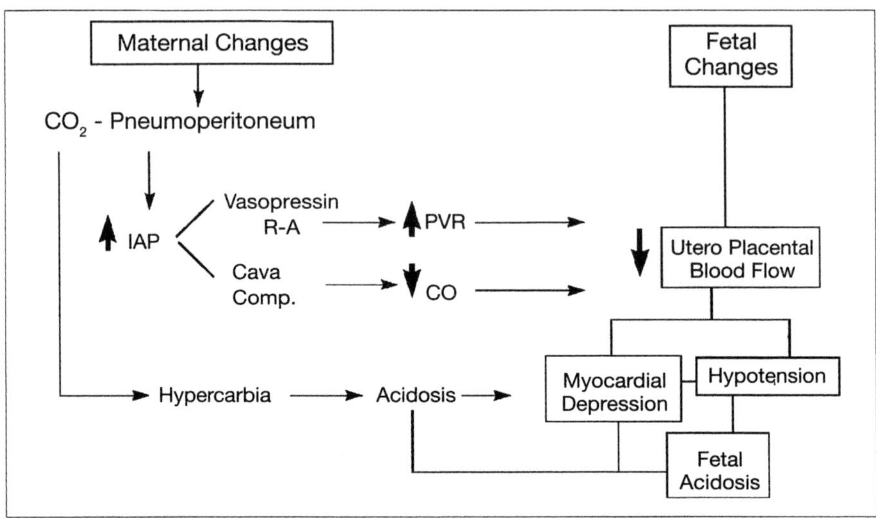

Fig. 3. Maternal and fetal changes in pneumoperitoneum during pregnancy. IAP, intra-abdominal pressure; R-A, *; PVR, pulmonary venous pressure; Comp., compression; CO, cardiac output

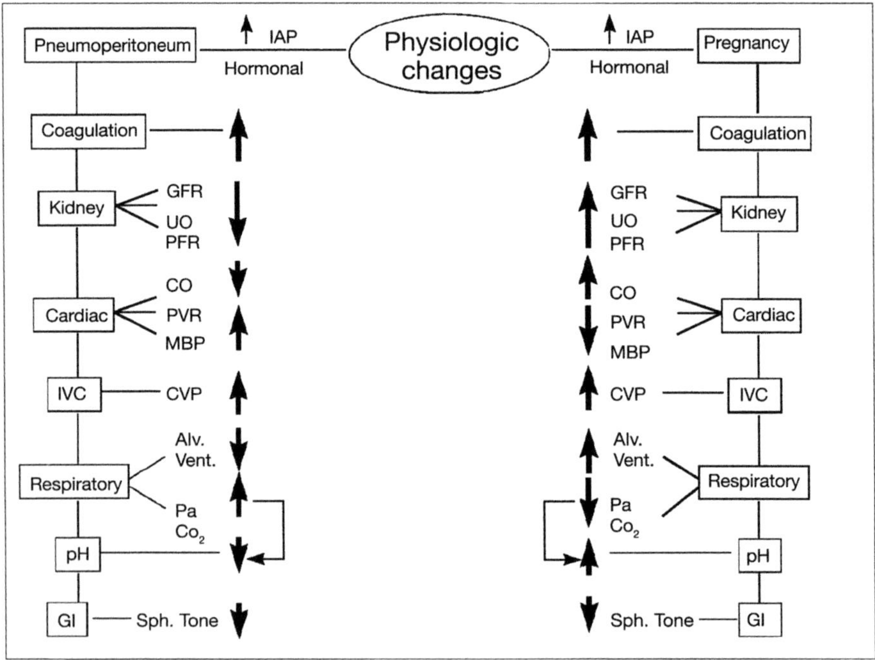

Fig. 4. Physiologic changes in pneumoperitoneum and pregnancy. IAP, intra-abdominal pressure; GFR, glomerular filtration rate; UO, *; PFR, *; CO, cardiac output; PVR, pulmonary venous pressure; MBP, mean blood pressure; IVC, inferior vena cava; CVP, *; Alv., alveolar; Vent., ventricular; GI, gastrointestinal; Sph., splanchnic;

and delivery. There is no indication for "elective" laparoscopic surgery during pregnancy.

The evaluation of gestational age, fetal heart tracing, and cervical dilation should be an integral part of the preoperative evaluation so that postoperative alterations in fetal growth, well-being, and uterine activity can be compared against a known baseline.

Positioning of the patient on her left side to avoid supine hypotension and its sequelae is important, in addition to the use of compression stockings with or without subcutaneous heparin to assist venous return and to prevent thromboembolic phenomena.

Limiting intra-abdominal pressures to the minimal necessary to effect adequate visualization and safe use of instruments, with close attention to maternal ventilation and acid–base status, is of utmost importance in minimizing the pathophysiologic consequences of pneumoperitoneum on the mother, and ultimately, the fetus.

As with any surgical patient, adequate hydration, careful monitoring of urine output, and aspiration precautions are paramount in the perioperative period.

Uterine manipulation should be avoided to minimize the risk of preterm labor. If necessary, however, tocolytic agents should be reserved for patients with significant preoperative uterine activity, documented cervical change, and/or risk of preterm delivery, determined for the most part by a prior history of preterm labor.

Intermittent fetal heart rate auscultation to document fetal life in the previable stage, and continuous monitoring at viability, with biophysical profile testing for nonreactive or nonreassuring tracings, is essential to follow fetal well-being. The decision to intervene for fetal distress should be made and prepared for in advance of the surgical procedure. Consultation with the neonatal team is integral in the planning of a possible emergent delivery, and in informing the prospective parents of survivability at the gestational age in question.

As with any intervention, the benefits must clearly outweigh the risks. In pregnancy, this is particularly important, for we are dealing with two patients. Careful preoperative assessment and selection of cases likely to benefit from laparoscopic surgery is essential, with the goal of optimizing the health and well-being of both the fetus and mother as the foremost concern. Simply being able to perform a procedure "through the scope" is not enough to subject all pregnant patients to laparoscopy. As popular as it may be, the available data are insufficient to draw conclusions regarding long term effects, if any, on the fetus. [4, 20] Until such effects are known, laparoscopy is best reserved for surgeons with extensive experience and expertise in performing these procedures in a carefully and wisely selected group of patients.

References

1. Allen JR, Helling TS, Langenfeld M (1989) Intra-abdominal surgery during pregnancy. Am J Surg 158:567–570
2. Barnard JM, Chaffin D, Droste S, Tierney A, Phernetton T (1995) Fetal response to carbon dioxide pneumoperitoneum in the pregnant ewe. Obstet Gynecol 85:669–674

3. Buss DD, Bisgard GE, Rawlings CA, Rankin JHG (1975) Uteroplacental blood flow during alkalosis in the sheep. Am J Physiol 228:1497–1500
4. CohenSE (1994) Nonobstetric surgery during pregnancy. In: Chestnut D (ed) Obstetric anesthesia principles and practice, 1st edn. Mosby, St. Louis, pp 273–293
5. Conklin KA (1994) Physiologic changes of pregnancy. In: Chestnut D (ed) Obstetric anesthesia principles and practice, 1st edn. Mosby, St. Louis, pp 17–42
6. Eisenach JC (1994) Uteroplacental blood flow. In: Chestnut D (ed) Obstetric anesthesia principles and practice, 1st edn. Mosby, St. Louis, pp 43–56
7. Freeman RK, Garite TJ, Naegeotte MP (1991) Fetal heart rate monitroing, 2nd edn. Williams and Wilkins, Baltimore
8. Guerrieri JP, Thomas RL (1994) Open laparoscopy for an adnexal mass in pregnancy. J Reprod Med 39:129–130
9. Harris A (1994) Fetal physiology. In: Chestnut D (ed) Obstetric anesthesia principles and practice, 1st edn. Mosby, St. Louis, pp 76–88
10. Kuller JA, Chesheir NC, Cefalo RC (1996) Prenatal diagnosis and reproductive genetics, 1st edn. Mosby, St. Louis, p 208
11. Lind T (1985) Maternal physiology basic science monograph in obstetrics and gynecology, 1st edn. Council on Resident Education in Obstetrics and Gynecology, Washington
12. Liu J, Feld RI, Goldberg BB, Barbot DJ, Nazarian LN, Merton DA, Rawool NM, Rosato FE, Winkel CA, Gillum DR et al (1995) Laparoscopic gray-scale and color Doppler US: preliminary animal and clinical studies. Radiology 194:851–857
13. Loughlin KR, Brooks DC (1992) The use of a Doppler probe to facilitate laparoscopic varicocele ligation. Surg Gynecol Obstet 174:326–328
14. Pucci RO, Seed RW (1991) Case report of laparoscopic cholecystectomy in the third trimester of pregnancy. Am J Obstet Gynecol 165:401–402
15. Punnonen R, Viinamaki O (1982) Vasopressin release during laparoscopy: role of increased intra-abdominal pressure. Lancet 1:175–176
16. RademakerBM, de Wit LT, Ringers J, Odoom JA (1991) Postoperative lung function and stress response after laparoscopic cholecystectomy. Anesthesiology 75:A123
17. Safran DB, Orlando R (1994) Physiologic effects of pneumoperitoneum. Am J Surg 167:281–286
18. Schreiber J (1990) Laparoscopic appendectomy in pregnancy. Surg Endo 4:100–102
19. Shalev E, Rahav D, Romano S (1990) Laparoscopic relief of adnexal torsion in early pregnancy. Case reports. Br J Obstet Gynecol 97:853–854
20. Soper N (1993) Effect of non biliary problems on laparoscopic cholecystectomy. Am J Surg 165:522–526
21. Weber AM, Bloom P, Allan TR, Curry SL (1991) Laparoscopic cholecystectomy during pregnancy. Obstet Gynecol 78:958–959

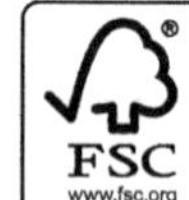

MIX
Papier aus verantwortungsvollen Quellen
Paper from responsible sources
FSC® C105338

If you have any concerns about our products,
you can contact us on
ProductSafety@springernature.com

In case Publisher is established outside the EU,
the EU authorized representative is:
Springer Nature Customer Service Center GmbH
Europaplatz 3, 69115 Heidelberg, Germany

Printed by Libri Plureos GmbH
in Hamburg, Germany